Understanding Violence Against Women

Nancy A. Crowell and Ann W. Burgess, editors

Panel on Research on Violence Against Women
Committee on Law and Justice
Commission on Behavioral and Social Sciences and Education
National Research Council

NATIONAL ACADEMY PRESS
Washington, D.C.   1996

NATIONAL ACADEMY PRESS • 2101 Constitution Avenue, N.W. • Washington, D.C. 20418

NOTICE: The project that is the subject of this report was approved by the Governing Board of the National Research Council, whose members are drawn from the councils of the National Academy of Sciences, the National Academy of Engineering, and the Institute of Medicine. The members of the committee responsible for the report were chosen for their special competencies and with regard for appropriate balance.

This report has been reviewed by a group other than the authors according to procedures approved by a Report Review Committee consisting of members of the National Academy of Sciences, the National Academy of Engineering, and the Institute of Medicine.

This project was supported under award # 95-IJ-CX-0006 from the National Institute of Justice, Office of Justice Programs, U.S. Department of Justice, and from the Centers for Disease Control and Prevention, U.S. Department of Health and Human Services. Points of view in this document are those of the authors and do not necessarily represent the official position of the U.S. Department of Justice or the U.S. Department of Health and Human Services.

Library of Congress Cataloging-in-Publication Data

Understanding violence against women / Panel on Research on Violence
    Against Women, Committee on Law and Justice, Commission on
    Behavioral and Social Sciences and Education, National Research
    Council.
        p.   cm
    Includes bibliographical references and index.
    ISBN 0-309-05425-7
    1. Women—Crimes against—United States. 2. Women—Crimes
    against—Research—United States. 3. Wife abuse—United States.
    4. Rape—United States. I. National Research Council (U.S.).
    Panel on Research on Violence Against Women. II. National Research
    Council (U.S.). Committee on Law and Justice. III. National
    Research Council (U.S.). Commission on Behavioral and Social
    Sciences and Education.
    HV6250.4.W65U53   1996
    362.82'92—dc20   96-17335
                                                                              CIP

Printed in the United States of America

Cover image by Photonica.

PANEL ON RESEARCH ON
VIOLENCE AGAINST WOMEN

ANN W. BURGESS (*Chair*), School of Nursing, University of
  Pennsylvania
EZRA C. DAVIDSON, JR. (*Vice Chair*), Department of Obstetrics
  and Gynecology, Charles R. Drew University of Medicine and
  Science, King-Drew Medical Center, Los Angeles
MARK APPELBAUM, Department of Psychology and Human
  Development, Vanderbilt University
LUCY BERLINER, Harborview Sexual Assault Center, Seattle
KIMBERLE CRENSHAW, Columbia University Law School
JEFFREY L. EDLESON, School of Social Work, University of
  Minnesota
DAVID A. FORD, Department of Sociology, Indiana University-
  Purdue University at Indianapolis
LUCY N. FRIEDMAN, Victim Services, New York
RICHARD B. IGLEHART, Office of the District Attorney,
  Alameda County Courthouse, Oakland, California
MARY P. KOSS, College of Medicine, University of Arizona
ILENA M. NORTON, National Center for American Indian and
  Alaska Native Mental Health Research, University of
  Colorado Health Services and Denver General Hospital
SUSAN B. SORENSON, School of Public Health, University of
  California, Los Angeles
SARA TORRES, Department of Community Nursing, University
  of North Carolina, Charlotte
ELIZABETH WATSON, Chief of Police, Austin (*to September
  1995*)
LINDA M. WILLIAMS, Family Research Laboratory, University of
  New Hampshire

NANCY A. CROWELL, *Study Director*
ROSEMARY CHALK, *Senior Project Officer*
KATHERINE DARKE, *Research Assistant* (from October 1995)
SEBLE MENKIR, *Research Assistant* (through July 1995)
NIANI SUTARDJO, *Project Assistant*

iii

Preface

Violence against women has received increasing public attention over the past 20 years. The once taboo subjects of rape and wife battering are now discussed openly on talk shows and are topics for television dramas. Services for women who have been raped or battered and men who rape and batter have become more available, although many services are chronically short of funds. Since the mid 1970s the body of research on violence against women has grown, yet misinformation abounds, and we seem little closer to ending violence against women now than 20 years ago.

The importance of violence against women as a national problem was acknowledged by Congress in its 1994 passage of the Violence Against Women Act as part of the Violent Crime Control and Law Enforcement Act and by President Clinton's establishment of an Office on Violence Against Women in the U.S. Department of Justice. The Panel on Research on Violence Against Women was established by the National Research Council in 1995 to fulfill a congressional request to develop a research agenda to increase the understanding and control of violence against women.

This report is the panel's response to that request. We have attempted to highlight the major literature on the scope of violence against women in the United States, the causes and consequences of that violence, and the interventions for both women victims of

violence and male perpetrators. The panel confined its deliberations primarily to rape, sexual assault, and battering of intimate
partners. Not only did the congressional request specifically mention rape and domestic violence as areas of interest, but also the
research base is larger on these topics than on others of potential
interest. For example, although panel members acknowledged concern over violence against women in the workplace, the research on
that topic is limited.

The panel was composed of members from a variety of disciplines, including nursing, gynecology-obstetrics, social work, law,
epidemiology, sociology, psychology, and psychiatry, as well as
methodologists. Some of the panel members have studied aspects
of sexual assault or domestic violence for most of their research
careers, some have expertise in related research fields, and some
have experience primarily in providing services. (See Appendix A
for biographical sketches of panel members and staff.)

With such diversity, disagreements were not uncommon. On
most issues, after discussion and literature reviews, consensus was
reached. The panel held lengthy discussions on defining violence
against women, focused on whether psychological abuse should be
included. The panel concluded that it could not resolve a question
that is still so open among researchers and that a global definition
was not necessary for carrying out our study. In our report we
discuss some of the controversies surrounding definitions, but do
not recommend a specific definition.

In carrying out its task, the panel met three times over the
course of 6 months to discuss research findings and gaps and needs
concerning violence against women. As part of its fact finding, the
panel also convened a workshop of researchers and practitioners.
(See Appendix B for the workshop topics and speakers.) The panel
thanks the workshop participants for sharing their expertise: our
work was enhanced by their presentations and the workshop discussions. The panel also gained insights from background papers on
violence against women in a lifespan perspective from Mary E.
Gilfus and on partner violence in lesbian relationships from Mary
Eaton.

The panel extends a special thanks to Mary Lieberman, head of
victim services for the Austin Police Department. She provided
great insights into the police perspective.

Each member of the panel contributed to the study by leading discussions, providing background readings, and reading and commenting on report drafts. Several members deserve special recognition for taking the lead in drafting report sections: Susan Sorenson—nature and scope; Mary Koss—causes and consequences; Jeffrey Edleson—interventions with batterers; David Ford—criminal justice system interventions; Lucy Berliner—treatment for sexual offenders; Ilena Norton—cultural sensitivity; Lucy Friedman—costs. The panel is indebted to study director Nancy Crowell for stitching these written contributions and the panel discussions into a report and to Eugenia Grohman, associate director for reports of the Commission on Behavioral and Social Sciences and Education, whose editorial skill vastly improved the report's organization and readability.

The panel extends sincere thanks to senior staff officer Rosemary Chalk for sharing her broad expertise in National Research Council committee process with the panel. The panel also extends its gratitude to project assistant Niani Sutardjo for her hard work setting up meetings, arranging travel, and preparing agenda materials. Research assistants Seble Menkir and Katherine Darke provided valuable assistance in locating background materials and checking references.

The panel is grateful for the support and patience of its sponsors and the interest of program officers Bernard Auchter of the National Institute of Justice and Pam McMahon of the Centers for Disease Control and Prevention.

Ann W. Burgess, *Chair*
Panel on Research on Violence
Against Women

The National Academy of Sciences is a private, nonprofit, self-perpetuating society of distinguished scholars engaged in scientific and engineering research, dedicated to the furtherance of science and technology and to their use for the general welfare. Upon the authority of the charter granted to it by the Congress in 1863, the Academy has a mandate that requires it to advise the federal government on scientific and technical matters. Dr. Bruce Alberts is president of the National Academy of Sciences.

The National Academy of Engineering was established in 1964, under the charter of the National Academy of Sciences, as a parallel organization of outstanding engineers. It is autonomous in its administration and in the selection of its members, sharing with the National Academy of Sciences the responsibility for advising the federal government. The National Academy of Engineering also sponsors engineering programs aimed at meeting national needs, encourages education and research, and recognizes the superior achievements of engineers. Dr. Harold Liebowitz is president of the National Academy of Engineering.

The Institute of Medicine was established in 1970 by the National Academy of Sciences to secure the services of eminent members of appropriate professions in the examination of policy matters pertaining to the health of the public. The Institute acts under the responsibility given to the National Academy of Sciences by its congressional charter to be an adviser to the federal government and, upon its own initiative, to identify issues of medical care, research, and education. Dr. Kenneth I. Shine is president of the Institute of Medicine.

The National Research Council was organized by the National Academy of Sciences in 1916 to associate the broad community of science and technology with the Academy's purposes of furthering knowledge and advising the federal government. Functioning in accordance with general policies determined by the Academy, the Council has become the principal operating agency of both the National Academy of Sciences and the National Academy of Engineering in providing services to the government, the public, and the scientific and engineering communities. The Council is administered jointly by both Academies and the Institute of Medicine. Dr. Bruce Alberts and Dr. Harold Liebowitz are chairman and vice chairman, respectively, of the National Research Council.

Contents

Understanding Violence Against Women

UNDERSTANDING VIOLENCE AGAINST WOMEN

ORDER CARD
(Customers in North America Only)

Use this card to order additional copies of UNDERSTANDING VIOLENCE AGAINST WOMEN and the book described on the reverse. All orders must be prepaid. Please add $4.00 for shipping and handling for the first copy ordered and $0.50 for each additional copy. If you live in CA, DC, FL, MD, MO, TX, or Canada, add applicable sales tax or GST. Prices apply only in the United States, Canada, and Mexico and are subject to change without notice.

___ I am enclosing a U.S. check or money order.

___ Please charge my VISA/MasterCard/American Express account.

Number: _____

Expiration date: _____

Signature: _____

Quantity Discounts:
5-24 copies   15%
25-499 copies   25%

To be eligible for a discount, all copies must be shipped and billed to one address.

Customers in North America Only: Return this card with your payment to NATIONAL ACADEMY PRESS, 2101 Constitution Avenue, NW, Lockbox 285, Washington, DC 20055. You may also order through your favorite bookstore, or electronically via Internet at http://www.nap.edu. All international customers please contact National Academy Press for export prices and ordering information.

PLEASE SEND ME:

Qty.	Code	Title	Price
___	VIOWOM	Understanding Violence . . . Women	$29.95
___	VIOLP	Understanding Violence, V1	$24.95
___	VIOL2	Understanding Violence, V2	$45.00
___	VIOL3	Understanding Violence, V3	$45.00
___	VIOL4	Understanding Violence, V4	$39.00
___	ABUSE	Understanding Child Abuse	$44.95
___	VIOURB	Violence in Urban Areas	$12.95

Please print.
Name _____

Address _____

City _____ State _____ Zip Code _____

To order by phone using VISA/MasterCard/American Express, call toll-free 1-800-624-6242 or call 202-334-3313 in the Washington metropolitan area. Fax 202-334-2451.

VIWC

Understanding Child Abuse and Neglect
ISBN 0-309-04889-3; 1993, 408 pages, 6 x 9, index, hardbound, $44.95

Understanding and Preventing Violence, Volume 1
ISBN 0-309-05476-1; 1993, 480 pages, 6 x 9, index, paperbound, $24.95

Understanding and Preventing Violence, Volume 2: Biobehavioral Influences
ISBN 0-309-04649-1; 1994, 568 pages, 6 x 9, paperbound, $45.00

Understanding and Preventing Violence, Volume 3: Social Influences
ISBN 0-309-05080-4; 1994, 592 pages, 6 x 9, paperbound, $45.00

Understanding and Preventing Violence, Volume 4: Consequences and Control
ISBN 0-309-05079-0; 1994, 408 pages, 6 x 9, paperbound, $39.00

Violence in Urban America: Mobilizing a Response
ISBN 0-309-05039-1; 1994, 118 pages, 6 x 9, paperbound, $12.95

Understanding Violence Against Women

Violence against women is one factor in the growing wave of alarm about violence in American society. High-profile cases such as the O.J. Simpson trial call attention to the thousands of lesser known but no less tragic situations in which women's lives are shattered by beatings or sexual assault. Understanding Violence Against Women presents a comprehensive overview of current knowledge and identifies four areas with the greatest potential return from a research investment by increasing the understanding of and responding to domestic violence and rape: What interventions are designed to do, to whom they are reaching, and how to reach the many victims who do not seek help? What factors put people at risk of violence and that precipitate violence? What is the scope of domestic violence and sexual assault in America and its consequences to individuals, families, and society? How should we structure the study of violence against women to yield more useful knowledge?

ISBN 0-309-05425-7; 1996, 240 pages, 6 x 9, index, hardbound, $29.95

Use the form on the reverse of this card to order your copies today.

Executive Summary

Violence against women is a major social problem in the United States. National surveys estimate that at least 2 million women each year are battered by an intimate partner, and crime data from the Federal Bureau of Investigation (FBI) record about 1,500 murders of women by husbands or boyfriends each year. Overall, the Bureau of Justice Statistics reports that women sustained about 3.8 million assaults and 500,000 rapes a year in 1992 and 1993: more than 75 percent of these violent acts were committed by someone known to the victim, and 29 percent of them were committed by an intimate—a husband, ex-husband, boyfriend, or ex-boyfriend. Studies estimate that between 13 and 25 percent of all U.S. women will experience rape in their lifetimes. These figures are believed to be underestimates.

The consequences of this violence against women may be long-lasting. Both rape and intimate partner violence (battering, which is frequently accompanied by psychological abuse) are associated with a host of both short- and long-term problems, including physical injury and illness, psychological symptoms, and, in extreme cases, death. And the conse-

1

quences go far beyond the individual female victims, affecting their children, families, and friends, as well as society at large.

Research on violence against women is a relatively young and fragmented field. At this early yet critical time in the developing field, Congress (in the Violence Against Women Act of 1994) directed the National Research Council to develop a research agenda to increase the understanding and control of violence against women, including rape and domestic violence. Congress specified that the agenda focus primarily on preventive, educational, social, and legal strategies, including consideration of the needs of underserved populations.

In convening the Panel on Research on Violence Against Women, the National Research Council specifically charged the panel with the following tasks: synthesize the relevant research literature and develop a framework for clarifying what is known about the nature and scope of violence against women; supplement the research review with lessons learned by field professionals and service providers; and identify promising areas of research to improve knowledge of the scope of the problem and interventions for dealing with it.

After reviewing the literature on battering, rape, and sexual assault, the panel concludes that significant gaps exist in understanding of the extent and causes of violence against women and the impact and effectiveness of preventive and treatment interventions. In order to begin filling those gaps, the panel recommends a research agenda to facilitate development in four major areas: preventing violence against women, improving research methods, building knowledge about violence against women, and developing the research infrastructure.

PREVENTING VIOLENCE AGAINST WOMEN

The panel concludes that in order to significantly reduce the amount of violence against women in the United States the focus must be on prevention. The development of effective preventive interventions will require a better understanding of the causes of violent behavior against women, as well as rigorous evaluations of preventive intervention programs. The panel, therefore, recommends:

- longitudinal research to study the developmental trajectory of violent behavior against women and whether and how it differs from the development of other violent behaviors;
- the inclusion of questions about violent behavior against women in research on the causes of other violent behavior;
- the examination of risk factors, such as poverty, childhood victimization, and brain injury, for sexual and intimate partner violence in studies of at-risk children and adolescents;
- rigorous evaluation of both short- and long-term effects of programs designed to prevent sexual and intimate partner violence, including school-based education programs, media campaigns, and legal changes intended to deter violence against women; and
- the inclusion of intimate partner and sexual violence outcomes in evaluations of nonviolent conflict resolution programs and other programs designed to prevent delinquency, substance abuse, teenage pregnancy, gang involvement, and general violence.

IMPROVING RESEARCH METHODS

Researchers working on violence against women come from a wide spectrum of disciplines, each of which has its own terms and perspectives. Many studies in the field suffer from methodological weaknesses, including small sample sizes, lack of control groups, and weak instrumentation.

The panel recommends several key topics for improving research on violence against women:

- clear definition by researchers and practitioners of the terms used in their work;
- the development and testing of scales and other tools of measurement to make operational the key and most used definitions;
- improvement in the reliability and validity of research instruments with guidance from subpopulations with whom the instruments will be used, for example, people of color or specific ethnic groups;
- clarification of theory and the outcomes expected from the intervention in evaluation research;
- the use of randomized, controlled outcome studies to identify the program and community features that account for effectiveness (or lack thereof) of legal and social service treatment interventions with various groups of offenders;
- both qualitative and quantitative research to recognize the confluence of the broad social and cultural context in which women experience violence, as well as individual factors, with attention to such factors as race, ethnicity, socioeconomic status, age, and sexual orientation in shaping the context and experience of violence in women's lives.

BUILDING KNOWLEDGE

There are many gaps in understanding of violence against women. There is relatively little information about violence against women of color, disabled women, lesbians, immigrant women, and institutionalized women. Research on violence against women has advanced along categorical lines (i.e., sexual violence, physical violence) rather than on women's experiences, which are believed to include multiple forms of violence. Although there appear to be some similarities and some differences between generally violent behavior and violence directed at women, the extent of the similarities and differences remains unknown.

The panel recommends the following areas as the most important next research steps:

- the development of both national and community-level survey studies using the most valid instrumentation and questioning techniques to measure incidence and prevalence of violence against women (both victimization and perpetration), with particular attention to surveys of racial and ethnic minorities, and other underrepresented population subgroups;
- the inclusion of questions pertaining to violence against women in national and community surveys of topics such as women's mental or physical health or social or economic well-being;
- identification and secondary analysis of existing data sets with respect to violence against women;
- research on the consequences of violence against women that includes intergenerational consequences, effects of race and socioeconomic status on consequences, and costs to society, including lost productivity and the use of the criminal justice, health, and social service systems;
- studies that describe current services for victims of violence and evaluate their effectiveness;
- studies to investigate the factors associated with victims' service-seeking behavior, including delaying seeking of services or not seeking services at all, in order to identify barriers to service seeking and alternative approaches and settings for service provision; and
- studies that examine discretionary processes in the criminal and civil justice systems, including legal research on the theory and implementation of new laws and reforms, police and prosecutorial decision making, jury decision making, and judicial decision making.

DEVELOPING THE RESEARCH INFRASTRUCTURE

Responsibility for research on violence against women is spread across a number of federal agencies, with most funding coming from the Centers for Disease Control and Prevention and the National Institutes of Health of the U.S. Department of Health and Human Services, and the National Institute of

Justice of the U.S. Department of Justice. A number of other agencies, including the National Science Foundation and the U.S. Department of Education, have programs that could contribute to the development of research on violence against women. The panel concludes that research on violence against women will be strengthened by a research infrastructure that supports interdisciplinary efforts and helps to integrate those efforts into service programs and institutional policies, especially in the area of preventive intervention.

The panel recommends two key actions for improving research capacity and strengthening ties between researchers and practitioners:

- development of a coordinated research strategy by government agencies; and
- establishment of a minimum of three to four research centers, within academic or other appropriate settings, to support the development of studies and training programs focused on violence against women, to provide mechanisms for collaboration between researchers and practitioners, and to provide technical assistance for integrating research into service provision.

The problem of violence against women in the United States will not be solved in the short term or without concentrated attention. Well-organized research will be critical to the long-term goal of preventing and ameliorating the effects of violence against women.

1

Introduction

Although men are more likely than women to be victims of violent crimes—61 per 1,000 for men, 42.6 per 1,000 for women (Bastian, 1995)—patterns of victimization differ. Women are far more likely than men to be victimized by an intimate partner (Kilpatrick et al., 1992; Bachman, 1994; Bachman and Saltzman, 1995). In fact, about three-quarters of all lone-offender violence against women in 1993 was perpetrated by someone known to the woman, compared with one-half of lone-offender violence against men (Bachman and Saltzman, 1995). It is important to note that attacks by intimates are more dangerous to women than attacks by strangers: 52 percent of the women victimized by an intimate sustain injuries, compared with 20 percent of those victimized by a stranger (Bachman and Saltzman, 1995). Women are also significantly more likely to be killed by an intimate than are men. In 1993, 29 percent of female homicide victims were killed by their husbands, ex-husbands, or boyfriends; only 3 percent of male homicide victims were killed by their wives, ex-wives, or girlfriends (Federal Bureau of Investigation, 1993).[1]

Women are more likely to be victimized by male offenders than by female offenders; about three-quarters of violent crimes against women are committed by males (Bachman, 1994). In one urban emergency room, violence was the most common cause of injury to women between the ages of 15 and 44 and the second most common cause of injury for all women (Grisso et al., 1991). Finally, women are far more likely than men to be sexually assaulted. The National Crime Victimization Survey (NCVS) found women were 10 times more likely to be raped or sexually assaulted than were men (Bastian, 1995). The annual rate of rape is estimated to be 7.1 per 1,000 adult women, and 13 percent of all women will experience forcible rape sometime during their lives (Kilpatrick et al., 1994).

The exact dimensions of violence against women are frequently disputed, yet even conservative estimates indicate that millions of American women experience violent victimization. The fear of violence, in particular the fear of rape, affects many more, if not most, women (Gordon and Riger, 1989). A few researchers have even suggested that learning to cope with the threat of violent victimization is a normative developmental task for females in the United States (Gilfus, 1995).

In spite of the attention that has been paid to violence against women in recent years, the research endeavor is relatively young, and much remains unknown. There really is no one field focused on violence against women per se. For example, studies on rape and sexual assault are distinct from those on intimate partner violence, which is distinct from the nascent study of stalking. And all this research is separate from that on violence in general. Many of the studies in this newly emerging field of research on violence against women are at an early stage of scientific rigor. The methodological weaknesses in the research on battering and rape have been discussed at length in other documents (Rosenbaum, 1988; Gelles, 1990; Koss, 1992, 1993; Rosenfeld, 1992; Smith, 1994). Definitions differ from study to study, making comparisons difficult. Much of the research on both victims and perpetrators is based on clinical samples, samples of convenience, or other nonrandomized samples, so one cannot draw general conclusions. Sample sizes are often quite small. Only recently have sophisticated statistical analyses been used. Yet in spite of all the shortcomings, a lot has been learned about the extent of violence against women, about perpetrators of violence, and about the effects on victims.

WHAT IS VIOLENCE AGAINST WOMEN?

The term violence against women has been used to describe a wide range of acts, including murder, rape and sexual assault, physical assault, emotional abuse, battering, stalking, prostitution, genital mutilation, sexual harassment, and pornography. There is little consensus in the still evolving field on exactly how to define violence against women. The major contention concerns whether to strictly define the word "violence" or to think of the phrase "violence against women" more broadly as aggressive behaviors that adversely and disproportionately affect women.

Researchers in such fields as sociology and criminology tend to prefer definitions that narrowly define violence, definitions that can be operationalized. For example, Gelles and Straus (1979) defined violence as "any act carried out with the intention of, or perceived intention of, causing physical pain or injury to another person." Similarly, the National Research Council (NRC) report *Understanding and Preventing Violence* (Reiss and Roth, 1993) limited its definition to "behavior by persons against persons that intentionally threatens, attempts, or actually inflicts physical harm." The 1993 NRC study deliberately excluded behavior that inflicts harm unintentionally, while the Gelles and Straus definition includes behaviors that may be unintentional but are perceived by the victim to be intentional. The 1993 NRC study also specifically excluded from its definition of violence such events as verbal abuse, harassment, or humiliation, in which psychological trauma is the sole harm to the victim. However, in its consideration of family violence and sexual assault, the report did include the psychological consequences of threatened physical injury.

In contrast to those definitions, researchers in such fields as psychology, mental health, and social work frequently consider "violence" to cover a wider range of behaviors. The Committee on Family Violence of the National Institute of Mental Health (1992) included in its definition of violence "acts that are physically and emotionally harmful or that carry the potential to cause physical harm . . . [and] may also include sexual coercion or assaults, physical intimidation, threats to kill or to harm, restraint of normal activities or freedom, and denial of access to resources." The Task Force on Male Violence Against Women of the American Psychological Association defined violence as "physical, visual, verbal, or sexual acts that are experienced by a woman or a girl as a threat, invasion, or assault and that have the effect of hurting her or degrading her and/or taking away her ability to control contact (intimate or otherwise) with another individual" (Koss et al., 1994). Those who argue for these broader definitions suggest they more accurately represent the experiences of victims, who often say they find verbal and psychological abuse more harmful than actual physical abuse (Walker, 1979; Follingstad et al., 1990; Herman, 1995).

In the field of intimate partner violence or battering, the problem of violence against women is frequently characterized as one of coercive control that is maintained by tactics such as physical violence, psychological abuse, sexual violence, and denial of resources. The concern is with the array of behaviors that are used to dominate women. Physical violence need not be used often to be effective: "In fact, abusers may regret resorting to violence, but may perceive themselves as 'driven to it' when their other methods of enforcing subordination are insufficient" (Herman, 1995:2). In the field of rape, fear is a key element; it is an overriding concern for many women (Warr, 1985; Gordon and Riger, 1989; Klodawsky and Lundy, 1994). Even though women are less frequently the victims of violent crime than men, women fear crime more (Federal Bureau of Investigation, 1991) and this fear appears to be largely based on their fear of rape (Riger et al., 1981). Many feminist theorists contend that this fear of rape serves to intimidate and control all women (e.g., Griffin, 1971; Brownmiller, 1975; Dworkin, 1991).

Although research would benefit from more unified definitions, the panel understands the difficulty of reaching agreement on definitional issues in light of the many complex behaviors that are involved. The panel held lengthy discussions on defining violence against women, focused on the key issue of whether psychological abuse should be included. The panel concluded that it could not resolve a question that is so open among researchers and that a global definition was not necessary for carrying out the task of reviewing what is known and recommending needed research (see below). Thus, the panel agreed that this study would be primarily a review of the literature on intimate partner violence (battering), rape, and sexual assault. The study does not include violence that occurs in conjunction with other crimes, such as robbery, burglary, or car theft. Nor does it include prostitution, sexual harassment, or issues such as genital mutilation, dowry murders, and trafficking in women that are more relevant internationally than in the United States.

Whether one uses a narrow definition confined to physical and sexual violence or one accepts a broader definition of violence against women, definitional debates also surround each of the individual components. For example, how does one define rape or sexual assault? Should all physical aggression or use of force be considered violent? What constitutes psychological abuse? These questions affect both the research that is done and how much it can be generalized.

Rape and Sexual Assault

Although all definitions of rape, sexual assault, and related terms include the notion of nonconsensual sexual behavior, the definitions used by researchers have varied along several dimensions. These include the behaviors specified, the criteria for nonconsent, the individuals involved, and who decides whether rape or sexual assault has occurred (Muehlenhard et al., 1992; Koss, 1993).

Many data sources and some researchers rely on legal definitions of rape, but those definitions differ from state to state and change over time. In common law, rape was traditionally defined as "carnal knowledge [penile-vaginal penetration only] of a female forcibly and against her will" (Bienen, 1980:174). The FBI's Uniform Crime Report (1993) still uses this narrow definition of rape even though most states have reformed their rape laws during the past 20 years. There have been three common reforms:

- broadening the definition to include sexual penetration of any type, including vaginal, anal, or oral penetration, whether by penis, fingers, or objects;
- focusing on the offender's behavior rather than the victim's resistance; and
- restricting the use of the victim's prior sexual conduct as evidence.

Many states have also removed the marital exemption from their rape laws. Some states and the U.S. Code (18 U.S.C. § 2241-2245) have replaced the term "rape" with terms such as "sexual assault," "sexual battery," or "sexual abuse" (Epstein and Langenbahn, 1994). Many laws now have a series of graded offenses defined by the presence or absence of aggravating conditions, making sexual assault laws similar to other assault laws. For example, the U.S. Code uses the categories aggravated sexual abuse when someone "knowingly causes another person to engage in a sexual act by using force against that other person, or by threatening or placing that other person in fear that any person will be subjected to death, serious bodily injury, or kidnapping" or by knowingly causing another person to become incapable of giving consent by rendering them unconscious or administering intoxicants. Sexual abuse involves lesser threats or engaging in sexual acts with a person who cannot give consent.

The definition of rape or sexual assault used in a research study has an effect on who is counted as a rape victim. The type of screening questions, the use of the word rape versus the use of behavioral descriptions, and other considerations all affect the research results (Koss et al., 1994). Higher rates of rape and sexual assault are found when behavioral descriptions and multiple questions are used than when surveys ask directly about rape or sexual assault. Women may not label experiences that meet the legal definition of rape or sexual assault as such, particularly if the perpetrator was an intimate partner or an acquaintance. The use of behavioral descriptions in studies assures that what is being measured are experiences rather than an individual's conceptions of the words rape or sexual assault.

In this report, rape means forced or coerced penetration— vaginal, anal, or oral; "sexual assault" means other forced or coerced sexual acts not involving penetration; and "sexual violence" includes both rape and sexual assault.

Physical Violence

Although defining physical violence would seem to be more clear-cut, there are disagreements both over definitions and measurement. As noted above, some researchers include only acts that were intended to cause physical harm or injury (Reiss and Roth, 1993); others argue that intentionality may be difficult to ascertain, and therefore physical violence should also include acts that are perceived as having the intention of producing physical harm or injury (Gelles and Straus, 1979). Akin to intentionality is the consideration of the context of the act. For example, should an action taken in self-defense be considered violent? Should an act be considered violent only if an injury occurs, or is the potential for injury sufficient? Some definitions of physical violence, following legal models of assault, include threats of physical harm; others consider that threats fall under verbal or psychological abuse (Straus, 1990a). There is disagreement about whether behaviors such as slapping a spouse should be equated with more severe acts such as kicking or using a weapon. How violence is defined and measured influences the rate of violence found in a study: all else being equal, the broader the definition, the higher the level of violence reported (Smith, 1994).

Physical violence is most commonly measured by the Conflict Tactic Scales (Straus, 1979, 1990b) or some modification of it. Such scales ask about the occurrence of various representative behaviors. For example, the Conflict Tactic Scales list nine physical violence items:

- threw something at you;
- pushed, grabbed, or shoved you;
- slapped you;
- kicked, bit, or hit you with a fist;
- hit or tried to hit you with something;
- beat you up;
- choked you;
- threatened you with a knife or gun; and
- used a knife or fired a gun.

The last six behaviors in this list are considered to be "severe" physical violence.

In this report, "physical violence" refers to behaviors that threaten, attempt, or actually inflict physical harm. The behaviors listed in the Conflict Tactic Scales, while not all inclusive, typify the type of behaviors meant by physical violence. In this report, "severe" violence refers to the type of behaviors typified by the severe violence items on the scales.

Psychological Abuse

Psychological abuse (also refered to as psychological maltreatment or emotional abuse) has received less research attention than physical or sexual violence, and hence there have been fewer attempts to define it. At a minimum, psychological abuse refers to psychological acts that cause psychological harm (McGee and Wolfe, 1991). It has been argued that separating physical and psychological conditions "overly simplifies the topic and denies reality" (Hart and Brassard, 1991:63): physically violent acts can have psychological consequences and psychological acts can have physical consequences. The difficulty of separating physical violence and psychological abuse is exemplified by the treatment of threats of physical violence, with researchers split over whether to classify such threats as physical violence or psychological abuse. As with physical violence, there is debate about intentionality; that is, must the offender intend harm for an act to be considered abuse? Deciphering the intention of a psychological act may be even more difficult than for a physical act, and so intention is generally not included in defining psychological abuse.

On the basis of descriptions of psychological abuse as reported by battered women, Follingstad et al. (1990) described the following categories of behavior as psychological abuse:

- verbal attacks such as ridicule, verbal harassment, and name calling, designed to make the woman believe she is not worthwhile in order to keep her under the control of the abuser;
- isolation that separates a woman from her social support networks or denies her access to finances and other resources, thus limiting her independence;
- extreme jealousy or possessiveness, such as excessive monitoring of her behavior, repeated accusations of infidelity, and controlling with whom she has contact;
- verbal threats of abuse, harm, or torture directed at the woman herself or at her family, children, or friends;

- repeated threats of abandonment, divorce, or of initiating an affair if the woman does not comply with the abuser's wishes; and
- damage or destruction of the woman's personal property.

Similar to measurements of physical violence, inventories or scales of representative behaviors are used to measure psychological abuse. The Conflict Tactics Scales subscale on verbal aggression (Straus and Gelles, 1990) measures some aspects of psychological abuse: items include "insulted or swore at you," "did or said something to spite you," "threatened to hit or throw something at you," and "threw or smashed or hit or kicked something." Other measures that have undergone validity testing are the Psychological Maltreatment of Women Inventory, which consists of 58 behavioral items (Tolman, 1988) and the Abusive Behavior Inventory, which includes items on both physical and psychological acts (Shepard and Campbell, 1992).

Interviews with battered women have detailed clear-cut examples of extreme psychological abuse occurring between and in conjunction with physically violent episodes. Psychological abuse frequently occurs with physical violence (Walker, 1979; Browne, 1987; Follingstad et al., 1990; Hart and Brassard, 1991), and research has repeatedly shown a strong association between psychological abuse and physical and sexual violence (e.g., O'Leary and Curley, 1986; Margolin et al., 1988; Sabourin et al., 1993). Some battered women describe psychological abuse—particularly ridicule—as constituting the most painful abuse they experienced (Martin, 1976; Walker, 1979, 1984; Follingstad et al., 1990). It has been suggested that ridicule may undermine a woman's self-worth, making her less able to cope with both physical violence and psychological abuse (Follingstad et al., 1990). Studies of child abuse have similarly shown that psychological maltreatment is present in most cases of physical abuse, and it predicts detrimental outcomes for children while severity of physical abuse does not (Claussen and Crittenden, 1991; Hart and Brassard, 1991).

In this report, "psychological abuse" refers to the types of behaviors described by Follingstad et al. (1990) and listed above, with the exception of threats of physical violence, which this report considers under physical violence. There is no separate section of the report devoted to psychological abuse because it has received very little study in and of itself. Rather, it is considered to be part of the pattern of behavior of serious physical violence, psychological abuse, and sometimes sexual violence, between intimate partners that has been well described (e.g., Martin, 1976; Dobash and Dobash, 1979; Walker, 1979; Browne, 1987). This pattern of behavior has been referred to in many terms, including domestic violence, spouse abuse, battering, and wife beating. "Wife beating" and "spouse abuse" imply married couples, although all intimate relationships—cohabiting, dating, and lesbian and gay couples—are frequently meant to be included under these terms. "Domestic violence," although usually referring to violence between intimate partners, is sometimes used to mean all forms of family violence, including child abuse, spouse abuse, sibling abuse, and elder abuse. These conflicting and overlapping terms and their uses are confusing in the study of violence against women.

In this report, "intimate partner violence" and "battering" are used synonymously to refer to the pattern of violent and abusive behaviors by intimate partners, that is, spouses, ex-spouses, boyfriends and girlfriends, and ex-boyfriends and ex-girlfriends.[2] The term batterer is used to mean the perpetrator of intimate partner violence, and battered woman, the victim.

In research studies, dating couples are sometimes considered as intimate partners and sometimes as acquaintances. "Acquaintance" generally refers to someone known to the victim but neither related nor an intimate. Particularly in crime data, it is not always clear what acquaintance means; it may include dating couples. Hence, date rape and dating violence are sometimes included in crime data as violence by nonintimate acquaintances.

Stalking

Battered women who have left their batterers have described being stalked by the batterer (e.g., Walker, 1979). This behavior includes following and threatening the woman, repeated harassing phone calls, threatening her family, and breaking into her living quarters. Anecdotal evidence suggests that some batterers go to extraordinary lengths to track down their victims and that women who are stalked by ex-partners may be at high risk of being killed. Although descriptive information about stalking is available, few data exist.

The acknowledgment of stalking as a crime is a fairly recent phenomenon. California passed the first antistalking law in 1990 (Sohn, 1994); today, 48 states and the District of Columbia have passed antistalking statutes (Boychuk, 1994). Most state statutes define stalking as willful, malicious, and repeated following and harassing of another person. Many statutes include in the definition the intent to place the victim in reasonable fear of sexual battery, bodily injury, or death.

THE PANEL'S CHARGE AND SCOPE

In the Violence Against Women Act of 1994 (Title IV of P.L. 103-322, the Violent Crime Control and Law Enforcement Act of 1994), Congress directed the National Research Council to develop a research agenda on violence against women (Chapter 9, § 40291):

> The Attorney General shall request the National Academy of Sciences, through its National Research Council, to enter into a contract to develop a research agenda to increase the understanding and control of violence against women, including rape and domestic violence. In furtherance of the

contract, the National Academy shall convene a panel of nationally recognized experts on violence against women, in the fields of law, medicine, criminal justice, and direct services to victims and experts on domestic violence in diverse, ethnic, social, and language minority communities and the social sciences. In setting the agenda, the Academy shall focus primarily on preventive, educative, social, and legal strategies, including addressing the needs of underserved populations.

In convening the Panel on Research on Violence Against Women, the National Research Council specifically charged the panel with the following tasks:

- synthesize the relevant research literature and develop a framework for clarifying what is known about the nature and scope of violence against women, including rape and domestic violence;
- supplement the research review with lessons learned by field professionals and service providers, including providers of services to ethnic, social, and language minorities; and
- identify promising areas of research to improve knowledge of the scope of the problem, and implementation and evaluation of preventive, educative, social, and legal interventions for dealing with violence against women.

In carrying out its charge, the panel limited its consideration to violence against women aged 12 and older. Child abuse and neglect and child sexual abuse were outside the purview of this panel and are covered by the report *Understanding Child Abuse and Neglect* (National Research Council, 1993), with a thorough research agenda.

The age of 12 was selected for several reasons. First, the types of violence to which teenage females are exposed are often more similar to violence directed at adult women than that directed at children. Second, sex offenders who prey on children seem to be quite different from those who target adolescent and adult women (Quinsey, 1984; Prentky, 1990).

Third, surveys on violence, such as The National Crime Victims Survey (NCVS), often include victims beginning at age 12. In addition, the highest rates of rape and sexual assault are found among women aged 12 to 24 years (Bachman and Saltzman, 1995): females in their teens and 20s are those most likely to be dating, and, therefore, subject to dating violence.

The panel's main task was to lay out a research agenda to improve understanding of violence and controlling that violence in the context of women's lives. This entailed reviewing the literature on intimate partner violence, rape, sexual assault, and stalking. The panel concentrated on studies published in peer-reviewed journals within the past 10 years, although very well-known or unique studies that were published earlier are also reviewed. The panel relied both on computerized literature searches, the expertise of various panel members, and monitoring a number of journals devoted to issues of violence. More than 300 journal articles and dozens of books were reviewed, many of which are cited in this report. The panel supplemented its literature review by holding a workshop of researchers and practitioners (see Appendix B).

The panel's review and analysis is divided into three topics: nature and scope, causes and consequences, and preventive and treatment interventions. Chapter 2 describes what the research shows about the nature and scope of violence against women. Chapter 3 discusses possible causes of violence against women and the consequences of violence to women and society. Chapter 4 examines preventive and treatment intervention efforts. Lastly, Chapter 5 discusses issues of research infrastructure and science policy on violence against women. Recommendations for research are discussed at the end of each chapter.

NOTES

1. The victim-offender relationship was not known in 39 percent of all homicides.

2. Although lesbian couples are technically included in this definition, there has been very little research on violence in lesbian (or male gay) relationships, and it is not covered separately in this report.

2
Nature and Scope of Violence Against Women

The problem of violence against women has gained increasing attention in recent years, but the scope and magnitude of the problem are the subjects of on-going debates (e.g., Gilbert, 1995). For example, studies of how many women experience rape in their lifetimes have reported as few as 2 percent (Riger and Gordon, 1981; Harris, 1993) and as many as 50 percent (Russell, 1984); most estimates fall between 13 and 25 percent (Koss and Oros, 1982; Hall and Flannery, 1984; Kilpatrick et al., 1987, 1992; Koss et al., 1987, 1991; Moore et al., 1989). There are similar debates about the number of battered women. Similar wide discrepancies are reported for women who experience violence by an intimate partner: annual rates range from 9.3 per 1,000 women (Bachman and Saltzman, 1995) to 220 per 1,000 women (Meredith et al., 1986). The most often cited figures come from the National Family Violence Surveys (Straus and Gelles, 1990), which found a rate of 116 per 1,000 women for a violent act by an intimate partner during the preceding year and 34 per 1,000 for "severe violence" by an intimate partner. The debates about scope and magnitude sometimes overshadow and divert attention from the discussion of the actual problem of violence against women, its consequences, and what can be done to prevent it.

This chapter highlights what is known about the extent of violence against women. It first reviews the data on the most extreme violence, that which ends in death. For nonfatal violence, the chapter considers information gathered from representative sample surveys and official data sources and discusses reasons for discrepancies in study findings. It also discusses gaps in the data, uses for data, and offers recommendations for improving the information about both the extent and nature of violence against women.

FATAL VIOLENCE

Data on homicides in the United States are collected by two sources—the Federal Bureau of Investigation (FBI) and the National Center for Health Statistics (NCHS). The FBI's Uniform Crime Reports (UCR) system collects basic information on serious crimes from participating police agencies and records supplemental information about the circumstances of homicides. The NCHS collects and tabulates data on causes of death, including homicide, from death certificates. The NCHS data provides detail on causes of death by homicide, by age, sex, and race, but it does not provide information on the offender-victim relationship.

Although U.S. homicide rates are substantially higher for men than for women—16.2 and 4.1 per 100,000, respectively (Federal Bureau of Investigation, 1993; Kochanek and Hudson, 1995)—homicide ranks similarly as a cause of death for both men and women; see Table 2.1. Homicide is the second leading cause of death for those aged 15-24 and the fourth leading cause for those aged 10-14 and 25-34. However, the pattern of offender-victim relationship for homicides has changed since the 1960s for men, but not for women. Today, men are more likely to be killed by a stranger or an unidentified assailant, while women are still substantially more likely to be killed

TABLE 2-1 Rank of homicide as a cause of death, by sex and age, 1990

Rank	Age of Victim								
	<1	1-4	5-9	10-14	15-19	20-24	25-34	35-44	45-54
1									
2					M, F	M, F			
3									
4				M, F			M, F		
5		M, F	M, F						
6									
7									
8								M	
9								F	
10	M, F								M

NOTE: Age categories for 55+ are not listed because homicide is not among the 10 leading causes of death for those ages. M, males; F, females.

SOURCE: Adapted from Sorenson and Saftlas (1994:141).

by a male intimate or an acquaintance (Mercy and Saltzman, 1989; Kellermann and Mercy, 1992; Federal Bureau of Investigation, 1993). In 1993, of the 4,869 female homicide victims (aged 10 and over), 1,531 (31 percent) were killed by husbands, ex-husbands, or boyfriends; of the 17,457 male homicide victims (aged 10 and over), only 591 (3 percent) were killed by wives, ex-wives, or girlfriends (Federal Bureau of Investigation, 1993). The rate of homicide by an intimate has remained remarkably stable for women, but not for men; see Figure 2.1. The rate for women was between 1.5 and 1.7 per 100,000 from 1977 to 1992. For men, however, the rate dropped from 1.5 per 100,000 in 1977 to 0.7 per 100,000 in 1992 (Bureau of Justice Statistics, 1994). It has been suggested that the availability of services for battered women, which began in the late 1970s, may have played a role in the decrease in males killed by intimates by offering women alternative means of escaping violent situations (see, e.g., Browne and Williams, 1989).

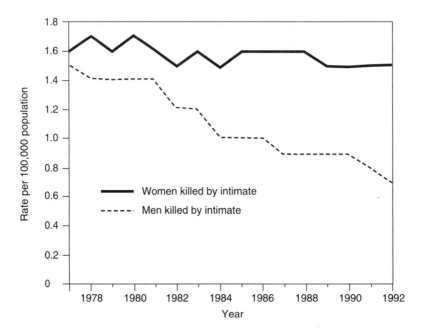

FIGURE 2-1 Rates of homicide by relationship to offender. NOTE: Intimate includes spouse, ex-spouse, and boyfriend or girlfriend. SOURCE: Bureau of Justice Statistics (1994:9)

Women, like men, are most likely to be murdered with a firearm (see, e.g., Kellermann and Mercy, 1992): 70 percent of all homicides in the United States in 1993 were committed with a firearm (Federal Bureau of Investigation, 1993). The risk of homicide in the home by a family member or intimate for both women and men is 7.8 times higher if a gun is kept in the home (Kellermann et al., 1993). Thus, laws that allow judges to require persons against whom temporary restraining orders (known also as protection-from-abuse orders) have been issued to relinquish firearms in their possession may help reduce the lethality of violence against women; the question has not yet been directly studied.

U.S. homicide rates are significantly higher for women of color than for white women: 10.7 per 100,000 for all women of color; 13.1 per 100,000 for African American women; 2.8 per 100,000 for white women (Kochanek and Hudson, 1995).

The same pattern holds for homicides by intimates. In 1992, the rate of intimate homicide of African American women aged 18 to 34 was 6 per 100,000; for whites in that age group the rate was 1.4 per 100,000 (Bureau of Justice Statistics, 1994).[1]

The overall homicide rate in the United States is 9.3 per 100,000 persons (Federal Bureau of Investigation, 1993), far higher than that of most other developed nations. For example, in Canada, a country that classifies most criminal offenses under rules similar to those in the United States, the 1993 homicide rate was slightly over 2 per 100,000. Interestingly, the homicide rate for Canadian women killed by their spouses is comparable to that in the United States, averaging 1.3 per 100,000 women each year; however, Canadian men are killed by their spouses at a rate of 0.4 per 100,000, about half the rate in the United States (Statistics Canada, 1994).

NONFATAL VIOLENCE

Official and Survey Data

Information on the scope of nonfatal violence against women comes from both official records and survey data. Thirty-five states collect some statistical information on domestic violence, and 30 states collect statistical data on sexual assaults (Justice Research and Statistics Association, 1996). However, the source and nature of the data vary greatly from state to state. Some states collect data from health or social service sources, such as hospital emergency rooms, other health care providers, or victim service provider records, but most of the data collected come from the criminal justice system, particularly from law enforcement agencies.

The Bureau of Justice Statistics of the Department of Justice and the Centers for Disease Control and Prevention of the Department of Health and Human Services have each funded demonstration projects to attempt to integrate data from the various sources to create a comprehensive data set on violence against women. While such data sets could be of great value to researchers and policy makers, concerns about confidentiality and the use of the data must be taken into account. For example, recording of domestic violence in women's medical records has resulted in some women being denied health insurance because domestic violence was classified as a preexisting condition.

The most consistently collected and commonly used official data set is the UCR. Because the FBI has been collecting and annually tabulating UCR data since 1930, they provide long-term, national trends. But the UCR includes only incidents that are considered crimes and that have been reported to the police. Based on comparisons with national survey data, it is estimated that only 40 to 50 percent of crimes become known to police (Reiss and Roth, 1993), and that percentages may be much lower for violent crimes against women. For example, a major survey of family violence found that only 6.7 percent of women assaulted by an intimate had reported the incident to police (Straus and Gelles, 1990). UCR rates further depend on the recording of reported incidents by the police as crimes. What is recorded may vary because of differences in state statutes (for example, marital rape would not be counted in those states in which it is not a crime), as well as by differences in policies among jurisdictions and the discretionary judgments of individual police officers. Furthermore, the UCR contains little information about nonfatal crimes other than race, age, and sex of arrested offenders; offender-victim relationship is not recorded.

In order to overcome the limitations inherent in official data, researchers have turned to surveys to gain a fuller picture of violence against women. Standard measures in survey research include incidence and prevalence. *Incidence* is the number of new cases within a specified time period (often, a year). *Prevalence* is the rate of established cases within a specified time period. Most of the surveys on violence against women measure either annual prevalence or lifetime prevalence (or both). Annual prevalence rates are important for looking at trends in the rate of violence over time; lifetime prevalence rates give an indication of the number of women who will be affected in the course of their lifetimes.

The primary sources for national data on violence against women are the two waves of the National Family Violence Survey (reported in Straus et al., 1980; Straus and Gelles, 1990), the on-going National Crime Victimization Survey,[2] and, for sexual assault, the National Women's Study (Kilpatrick et al., 1992). A number of other studies have addressed a distinct subpopulation or specific topic. Table 2.2 lists representative studies, their characteristics, and their findings.

Many of the studies on sexual assault cited in Table 2.2 were funded by the National Center for the Prevention and Control of Rape, which was located in the National Institute of Mental Health from 1976 until its termination in 1987. Currently, both foundation and federal government funding sources emphasize ameliorating the aftereffects rather than assessing the nature and scope of violence against women. Overall, there have been few survey studies on violence against women, and methodological constraints have precluded direct comparison across investigations, yet few resources in either the public or private sector are currently available for such work.

Research Findings

The more than 20 years of survey research on violence against women show a number of consistent patterns. The most common assailant is a man known to the woman, often her male intimate. This holds true for both sexual (e.g., Russell, 1982; Bachman and Saltzman, 1995) and physical (e.g., Kellermann and Mercy, 1992) assault. It also holds true for African Americans (e.g., Wyatt, 1992), Mexican Americans (e.g., Sorenson and Telles, 1991), and whites (e.g., Russell, 1982) and for both urban (e.g., Russell, 1982; Wyatt, 1992) and rural (e.g., George et al., 1992) populations.

TABLE 2-2 Representative sample studies of violence against women in the United States

Author(s) and Year	Sample	Ethnic composition	Locale	Findings
Sexual Assault				
Russell, 1982	930 adult women	Representative of area population	San Francisco	Lifetime rape reported by 24%
Hall and Flannery, 1984	508 adolescents (age 14-17)	—[a]	Milwaukee	Lifetime rape or sexual assault reported by 12%
Essock-Vitale and McGuire, 1985	300 women, 35-45 years old	100% white	Los Angeles	Lifetime rape or molestation reported by 22%
Kilpatrick et al., 1985	2,004 adult women	66% white 44% nonwhite[b]	Charleston County, SC	Lifetime forcible rape reported by 8.8%
Sorenson et al., 1987	1,645 women, 18-39 years old 1,480 adult men	6% Hispanic 42% non-Hispanic white, 13% other	Los Angeles	Lifetime sexual assault reported by 10.3% of Hispanic women, 26.3 % of non-Hispanic white women and 10% of all men
Wyatt, 1992	248 women, 18-36 years old	50% African American 50% white	Los Angeles	Rape since age of 18 reported by 25% of African American and 20% of white women

Study	Sample	Representativeness	Location	Findings
Kilpatrick et al., 1992	4,008 adult women	—[a]	United States	Lifetime rape reported by 13%
George et al., 1992	1,157 adult women	60.3% white 39.7% African American	Five counties in North Carolina	Lifetime sexual assault reported by 5.9%
Physical Assault by Intimate Partner				
Straus et al., 1980: National Family Violence Survey, 1975	2,146 adults	Representative of U.S. population	United States	Past year physical violence reported by 12.1% of women; past year severe violence reported by 3.8% of women
Schulman, 1979	1,793 adult women	Representative of state	Kentucky	Past year physical violence reported by 10%; ever experienced physical violence reported by 21%
Straus and Gelles, 1990: National Family Violence Survey, 1985	6,002 households	Representative of U.S. population	United States	Past year physical violence reported by 11.6% of women; past year severe violence reported by 3.4% of women

[a]Information not reported in study.

[b]Most nonwhite sample members were African American, with not more than 1% accounting for any other racial classification (e.g., Hispanic, American Indian, or Asian).

The highest rates of violence are experienced by young women. The average annual rate of victimization is 74.6 per 1,000 for women aged 12-18 and 63.7 per 1,000 for women aged 19-29; in comparison, the average annual rate for all women is 36.1 (Bachman and Saltzman, 1995). Although the actual rates may vary, the age trend is similar for homicides (Federal Bureau of Investigation, 1993), sexual assaults (Kilpatrick et al., 1992), and intimate partner violence (e.g., Straus and Gelles, 1990).

Women self-report violent actions toward their male partners at rates similar to or higher than men self-report violent actions toward their female partners (e.g., Straus and Gelles, 1986). However, men consistently have been found to report their own use of violence as less frequent and less severe than their female partners report it to be (Szinovacz, 1983; Jouriles and O'Leary, 1985; Edleson and Brygger, 1986; Fagan and Browne, 1994). Furthermore, rates do not provide information on the outcome of the act or whether the violent act was one of self-defense or attack, so the meaning of this finding is unclear. Both survey findings and health and crime data do indicate, however, that women are more frequently and more seriously injured by intimates than are men (Langan and Innes, 1986; Stets and Straus, 1990; Browne, 1993; Fagan and Browne, 1994).

Differences in study findings are primarily ones of magnitude rather than substance. For example, although risk characteristics (e.g., being young) and assault characteristics (e.g., by a known man) are fairly consistent across studies, estimates of the lifetime prevalence of sexual assault range from 2 percent (Riger and Gordon, 1981) to 50 percent (Russell, 1984) with most estimates hovering around 20 percent (e.g., Brickman and Briere, 1984; Essock-Vitale and McGuire, 1985). There have been so few representative sample investigations of physical violence against women that cross-study comparisons are necessarily limited. The 1992-1993 National Crime Victimization Survey (NCVS) found 34.7 of every 1,000 women had been victims of assault in a year: 8 per 1,000 for aggravated assault and 26.7 per 1,000 for simple assault, with 7.6 per 1,000 being assaults by intimates (Bachman and Saltzman, 1995). In contrast, in the 1985 National Family Violence Survey (NFVS) 116 women per 1,000 reported being victims of violence by an intimate (Straus and Gelles, 1990). The huge difference between the NFVS and the NCVS rates of assaults on women by intimates—the NFVS rate is 15 times higher—has been attributed to the difference in contexts of the two surveys: the NCVS questions relate to crimes; women may not view assaults by intimates as criminal, hence fail to report them in this context (Straus and Gelles, 1990).

Few data are available to determine how violence against women has changed over time or how it is related to overall rates of violence. In the United States, the rate of reported violent crime has increased dramatically in the past 20 years, from 46.1 per 1,000 in 1974 to 74.6 per 1,000 in 1993—a 61.8 percent increase (Federal Bureau of Investigation, 1993). In that same time span, the rate of forcible rape reported to police increased 54.9 percent (Federal Bureau of Investigation, 1993), but is not known how much of that increase may reflect increased willingness of women to report rape to the police and how much is an actual increase in the rate of rape. From 1973 to 1991, the rate of overall violence against women remained relatively constant at about 23 per 1,000 (Bachman, 1994). The NCVS did not specifically ask about sexual assaults or violence by intimates prior to 1992; after changes in the survey to specifically include such information, the reported rates of violence jumped to 43.7 per 1,000 women (Bachman and Saltzman, 1995). This change most likely reflects the change in the survey and not a sudden increase in the rate of violence against women. The NFVS found a 6.6 percent drop in the rate of intimate violence against women from the 1975 survey to the 1985 survey, although the drop was not statistically significant. In addition, the 1975 survey was conducted by face-to-face interviews and the 1985 survey was conducted by telephone: this difference may account for some of the drop in reported rates.

Although the United States has significantly higher rates of most violent crimes than most other developed countries (Reiss and Roth, 1993), rates of violence against women may be more similar. Table 2.3 shows the results of random sample surveys in a number of countries. The recent Canadian Violence Against Women Survey found that 29 percent of ever-married women had experienced physical or sexual violence at the hands of an intimate partner; in comparison, Straus and Gelles (1986) estimated that violence occurred in 28 percent of marriages in the United States. The Canadian survey also found that nearly 50 percent of all Canadian women had experienced at least one incident of physical or sexual assault since the age of 16 (Statistics Canada, 1994). The Canadian survey is remarkable in that it interviewed a random sample of 12,300 women who were 18 years of age and older and investigated physical and sexual violence as well as emotional abuse.

Accounting for Differences in Findings

As with all research, a variety of methodological factors can be linked to the differences in study findings. Sample composition and locale, data collection method, and question construction and context are among the most important methodological differences in U.S. studies.

Study samples vary widely. Although some include large numbers of African Americans (George et al., 1992; Wyatt, 1992) or Hispanics[3] (Sorenson et al., 1987; Kantor et al., 1994), most focus on European American (white) populations. With a few exceptions (e.g., George et al., 1992), most studies were conducted with urban residents. Given differences in the geographic location, age, and ethnic composition of the samples, one would not expect similar prevalence estimates.

Data collection methods also vary across the studies. Paper-and-pencil self-report instruments, once thought to be preferable because they allow for anonymity, have the lowest participation rates and produce the lowest prevalence estimates of adult sexual assault (Brickman and Briere, 1984; Hall and Flannery, 1984). Telephone interviews have been shown to be a substantial improvement over paper-and-pencil surveys because some rapport between the interviewer and the woman can be established and because more detailed and specific information can be collected. Face-to-face interviews, the most costly data collection method, are generally preferred for the investigation of sensitive topics, such as violence in intimate relationships, because they allow for the greatest interviewer-respondent rapport. Sexual assault prevalence rates obtained in studies that gathered data through in-person interviews are generally higher than those obtained in telephone interviews; those rates, in turn, are generally higher than the rates obtained in paper-and-pencil surveys (Russell, 1982; Hall and Flannery, 1984; Kilpatrick et al., 1985; Wyatt, 1992).

Definitions of violence against women vary from study to study. Some studies of sexual assault were limited to rape (e.g., Essock-Vitale and McGuire, 1985); others included physical contact in addition to rape (e.g., Wyatt, 1992); and still others used a very broad definition that included non-contact abuse (e.g., Sorenson et al., 1987). Given the discrepancy in definitions used to assess the phenomenon, differences in prevalence rates are to be expected.

Multiple, behaviorally specific questions are associated with greater disclosure by study participants. Studies of sexual assault that use a single screening question (e.g., "Have you ever been raped or sexually assaulted?") no matter how broad it is (e.g., Sorenson et al., 1987) obtain lower prevalence rates than studies that use several questions that are behaviorally specific (e.g., "Did he insert his penis into your vagina?") (e.g., Wyatt, 1992). Asking directly about sexual violence does not appear to offend study participants. In one community-based survey (Sorenson et al., 1987), a number of respondents talked about their assaults for the first time when responding to a direct question by the interviewer. Also, consistent with decades of social science research that docu-

TABLE 2-3 Representative sample studies of violence against women in other countries

Country and Author(s)	Sample	Sample Type	Findings
Barbados Handwerker, 1993	264 women aged 20-45 243 men aged 20-45	Islandwide national probability sample	30% of women battered as adults
Belguim Bruynooghe et al., 1989	956 women aged 30-40	Random sample of 62 municipalities	3% experienced serious; violence; 13% experienced moderately serious violence; 25% experienced less serious violence
Canada Statistics Canada, 1993	12,300 women over age 18	Random national sample	25% of women (29% of ever-married women) experienced physical or sexual violence by a male partner
Canada Brickman and Briere, 1984	551 adult women	Representative of city of Winnipeg	6% experienced rape and 21% sexual assault
Chile Larrain, 1993	1,000 women aged 22-55	Stratified random sample in Santiago	60% experienced abuse by male intimate; 26% experienced severe violence in relationship for at least 2 years

Colombia PROFAMILIA, 1990	3,272 urban women 2,118 rural women	National random sample	20% physically abused 33% psychologically abused 10% raped by husband
Korea, Republic of Kim and Cho, 1992	707 women and 609 men who had been with partner at least 2 years	Three-stage, stratified random sample of entire country	37.5% of wives report being battered by husband in past year
Malaysia Women's AID Organization, 1992	713 women over age 15 508 men over age 15	National random sample of peninsular Malaysia	39% of women physically beaten by a partner in 1989
New Zealand Mullen et al., 1988	349 women	Stratified random sample selected from electoral rolls of five contiguous parliamentary constituencies	20% physically abused by partner
Norway Schei and Bakketeig, 1989	150 women aged 20-49	Random sample selected from census data in Trondheim	25% physically or sexually abused by male partner

SOURCE: Adapted from Heise et al. (1994:6-9).

ments similar patterns with regard to sensitive topics, respondents in surveys were more likely to refuse to answer questions about income than they were to refuse to answer questions about sexual assault.

Prevalence estimates are also related to the context in which questions about sexual or intimate partner violence are asked. For example, the NCVS recently was amended to ask directly about sexual assault. Although such a change is an improvement over previous NCVS practice (to clearly define events such as robbery and burglary but not to name or directly ask about sexual assault), asking about sexual or intimate partner violence in the context of a survey about crime requires the respondent to define her experience as a criminal act (e.g., Koss, 1992). Research consistently shows, however, that women often do not define experiences that meet the legal definition of a rape as a rape (e.g., Koss, 1988), so they may be unlikely to respond affirmatively to questions about sexual assault that are asked in the context of a survey about criminal acts.

The context of the data collection is important in another way: women are known to be less likely to reveal incidents involving their male intimates, a common assailant according to survey research. There are a number of reasons for this phenomenon. Women may believe assaults by an intimate are family matters that should not be disclosed; they may fear losing their children should the violence become known; they may have concerns about involving the criminal justice system if the violence becomes known; and their assailants may be nearby at the time of the interview.

Like investigations into other sensitive topics (e.g., child sexual abuse; see Wyatt and Peters, 1986), most investigations have tried to reduce the differences between interviewers and study participants. One study that included both male and female interviewers and male and female respondents (Sorenson et al., 1987) found that the sex of the interviewer had little effect on prevalence estimates. Responses may vary on more subtle matters, however, and the issue of interviewer-respondent similarity on sociodemographic characteristics, such as gender and race, has not been deeply investigated.

Using the Available Data

Policy decisions—such as how many resources to allocate to service delivery—require solid data about the incidence and prevalence of violence against women. Rather than viewing the discrepancies in prevalence estimates as a problem, the range of findings may be very useful to decision makers. For example, differing estimates on the prevalance of sexual assault research results that are related to methodological differences, can be used for different pupuses. Research investigations that ask directly about sexual assault (and which obtain relatively low prevalence rates) ascertain the number of women who are willing to label themselves as survivors or victims of sexual assault and, therefore, who might seek sexual assault services. At the same time, it is important to estimate the number of women whose experiences are legally defined as sexual assault although they themselves might not define them that way: research indicates that those women use health services more frequently than women who have not been sexually assaulted, even when their health status and health insurance coverage are nearly identical (Koss et al., 1991). Thus, the "true" prevalence of violence against women may be less important for policy and other decision makers than understanding the methodological differences that resulted in various estimates.

Recognizing the commonalities in study findings of various investigations is critical to both policy and research. Research consistently documents that men known to women are those most likely to assault them (whether physically or sexually) and that young women are at high risk. These consistent findings suggest that scarce resources designated for men's violence against women should be allocated not to "stranger danger," but to the problem of violence by intimates and acquaintances. The research indicates the relative importance of preventing violence against young women.

Data Gaps

Although some policy decisions can be based on existing research, improving estimates of the rates of violence against women is important for a number of reasons. Without solid baseline rates for the general population and for various groups within the population, it is difficult to assess the effectiveness of interventions, particularly preventive interventions and interventions aimed at community-wide change. Good incidence and prevalence data—though they may measure different phenomena—are also important for the allocation of service resources. A number of substantial gaps exist in the knowledge base.

First, there is relatively little information about violence against a growing segment of the nation's population—women of color. Second, research on violence against women has advanced knowledge along categorical lines (i.e., sexual assault, physical assault) rather than on what are believed to be patterns of victimizaiton that include multiple forms of violence (e.g., Yoshihama and Sorenson, 1994). Third, studies have focused primarily on the victims, not the offenders, so there is little information on rates of perpetration. Estimates can be made of the number of women likely to experience sexual assault or intimate violence at sometime in their lives, but there is a lack of data with which to estimate the lifetime prevalence of violence perpetration. The scope of perpetration has implications for designing preventive interventions.

The studies conducted to date present a complex picture of ethnic differences in violence against women (Sorenson, 1996). National survey studies suggest that African Americans are more likely than white Americans to report physical violence in an intimate relationship (Straus and Gelles, 1986; Cazenave and Straus, 1990; Hampton and Gelles, 1994; Sorenson et al., 1996). However, how much of the variance may be explained by socioeconomic factors and how much by cultural factors remains unclear and requires further study. Studies that included Hispanics showed contradictory conclusions. Hispanics were reported to be at higher (Straus and Smith, 1990), similar (Sorenson and Telles, 1991), or lower (Sorenson et al., 1996) risk than non-Hispanic whites for physical violence in marriage. It is possible that this range of findings is due to sample differences, study contexts, and different data collection methods. It is also important to consider intragroup differences: for example, one study of four Hispanic groups—Puerto Rican, Mexican, Mexican-American, and Cuban—found prevalence rates for wife assault varied among them (Kantor et al., 1994). In-person interviews with representative samples of women reveal little difference in sexual assault prevalence between African American and white women (George et al., 1992; Wyatt, 1992). By contrast, unlike the findings for physical violence, studies have found Hispanic women (mostly of Mexican descent) to be at significantly lower risk of sexual assault than their non-Hispanic white counterparts (Sorenson et al., 1987; Sorenson and Telles, 1991). However, a substantial and consistent proportion of sexual assaults, regardless of respondent ethnicity, are perpetrated by the woman's male intimate (Sorenson et al., 1987; Sorenson and Telles, 1991; George et al., 1992; Wyatt, 1992).

There are no survey studies, to the panel's knowledge, of Asian American women's experiences of intimate violence. Such research is important because, according to Ho (1990: 129): "traditional Asian values of close family ties, harmony, and order may not discourage physical and verbal abuse in the privacy of one's home; these values may only support the minimization and hiding of such problems." Moreover, we have few data on different Asian and Pacific Islander populations, despite prevailing differences among these subgroups in terms of culture, value systems, immigration history, and other factors.

There is also limited information on the prevalence of

violence against women in American Indian and Alaska Native communities. There may be significant intertribal differences with the tremendous diversity in tribal cultures and over 250 recognized tribes, 209 Alaska Native villages, and 65 communities not recognized by the federal government (Norton and Manson, 1996). There are reports that domestic violence was rare, at least in some tribes, prior to contact with Europeans (Chester et al., 1994). It is possible that traditional family structures and social and religious functions may have served as protective factors.

Recent immigrants often are not represented in survey samples because of language and cultural barriers, immigrants' fears of officials and deportation, and fear that applications for relatives to immigrate to the United States might be affected (Chin, 1994). One study that examined immigrant status (i.e., whether the respondent was born in the United States) in association to physical or sexual assault by intimates offered surveys in either Spanish or English and found that persons born in Mexico evidenced a much lower risk of both physical and sexual violence in their intimate relationships than their U.S.-born Hispanic counterparts (Sorenson and Telles, 1991). These differences in risk patterns were not identified in two other studies of Latinos (Straus and Smith, 1990; Sorenson et al., 1996), in no small part because relatively recent immigrants were not likely to have been sampled since neither of these latter two studies interviewed anyone in Spanish. Diversity in the primary variable of interest, culture, is attenuated when monolingual non-English speaking populations are excluded.

There is a further methodological problem. Most studies have used measures and instruments developed on Anglos and simply applied them to members of other ethnic groups, for whom the instruments' validity is unknown. There may be differences in the intent of a question and a respondent's interpretation related to patterns of expression and idioms that may vary across cultures. This may explain, in part, the lack of consistency of results across studies. Clearly, unique cultural manifestations of violence against women cannot be identified if such experiences are not measured. The failure to include women of color in the development of instruments designed to assess violence against women has left the field with a major gap in the data.

In addition to data gaps about the prevalence of violence among minority women, there is also little conceptual understanding of how structural factors relating to race or ethnicity and socioeconomic status interact with gender to create the specific context in which violence is experienced (Crenshaw, 1991). These conceptual gaps can sometimes lead to oversights and omissions that can lead to policies that unintentionally exacerbate some women's vulnerability to violence. For example, immigration policies that required immigrant women to remain married to a resident spouse for 2 years before they could receive permanent residence status forced some women to remain in violent situations. Although there is anecdotal evidence that language barriers, immigrant status, geographical or social isolation, and cultural insularity can influence the experience of violence and the accessibility of interventions, these dynamics have not been systematically researched.

Additionally, there is little systematic information about the intersection of different forms of violence. One could speculate that a woman who is beaten by her husband on a regular basis is likely to be sexually victimized and psychologically maltreated as well, but survey research seldom investigates the co-occurrence of various forms of violence against women. Most surveys have focused on single aspects of women's experiences of violence, such as rape or physical violence. For example, studies of intimate partner violence that neglect to ask about sexual violence may miss information on and understanding of marital rape. Case studies of battered women indicate that the most severely battered women also experience severe sexual violence (Browne, 1987).

Another source of data may be studies of women's health and behavior that include unanalyzed information pertinent to violence against women. Identification and secondary analysis of these types of data sets could yield much information and at a relatively low cost. The inclusion of research questions pertaining to violence against women in other studies, such as those pertaining to women's health, alcohol and drug use, prenatal care, or unplanned pregnancy, could further help illuminate the context in which women experience violence and its impact on their lives. For example, existing health surveys could be amended to include questions about violence in women's lives. Research suggests that pregnant women who are battered are more likely to delay obtaining prenatal care (McFarlane et al., 1992) and to have low birthweight babies (Bullock and McFarlane, 1989) than pregnant women who are not battered. Cigarette smoking, alcohol and other drug intake, mental health status, and other relatively sensitive topics have been investigated in numerous studies of pregnancy. Including questions about being hit, kicked, or otherwise injured by one's male intimate may yield key information for understanding of pregnancy complications and outcomes, as well as of violence itself. Physical and sexual violence may account for some of the unexplained factors in women's health status that have been noted.

CONCLUSIONS AND RECOMMENDATIONS

Violence against women has been recognized as an important field of scientific inquiry, and the research to date has illuminated many aspects of women's experiences with violence. However, that research has often been narrowly focused, and comparisons across studies have been hampered by methodological differences.

Definitions and Measurement

Research definitions of violence against women have been inconsistent, not only making study findings difficult to compare, but also contributing to controversy over the scope of the problem. More consistent definitions and improved measures covering all aspects of violence against women would facilitate needed research on violence against women and improve knowledge as a basis for both research and policy.

Recommendation: Researchers and practitioners should more clearly define the terms used in their work.

Researchers, policy makers, and service providers from a wide spectrum of disciplines and fields—including public health, criminal justice, medicine, sociology, social work, psychology, and law—work on violence against women, and they need to ensure that others can understand and use their findings. The definitions need to take into account the full range of abuse experienced by women—sexual, physical, and psychological—and acknowledge the commonalities among, as well as unique aspects of, those forms of violence. Definitions that take into account the multidimensional aspects of violence against women will allow for the assessment of multiple types of violence against women in the same sample. Definitions should also specify severity, duration, and frequency of violent acts.

Recommendation: Research funds should be made available for the development and validation of scales and other tools for the measurement of violence against women to make operational key and most used definitions. The development process should include input from subpopulations with whom the instrument will be used, for example, people of color or specific ethnic groups.

There has been much controversy in the field over instruments used to measure violence against women, and the paucity of validated instruments is a serious barrier to improved research on violence against women. The context in which questions are asked and the wording used may influence the willingness of respondents to report violence. The context and wording of questions may also have different meanings for different subpopulations. In fields in which few measurement instruments are available, determining construct validity (the extent to which the association between a measure and other variables is consistent with theoretical or empirical knowledge) and concurrent validity (the extent to which a measure is related to other presumably valid measures) may be difficult. Repeated use and refinement of the test instrument, with careful attention to such aspects of measurement as format, administration conditions, and language level, may be necessary. Instrument developers may receive guidance on validity determination from the *Standards for Educational and Psychological Testing* (American Eduational Research Association et al., 1995).[4]

After work on instrumentation, including investigations of effective questioning strategies in relevant subpopulations, funding is needed for survey studies of varying sizes and scope (including different age groups and ethnic or racial groups) to rigorously document the extent of violence against women. Although some national surveys have estimated the frequency of violence against women, few national lifetime prevalence data exist, especially for racial and ethnic subgroups and other subpopulations. Because most surveys include persons who have experienced violence and sought services, those who have experienced violence but not sought services, and those who have not experienced violence, they can investigate the range of experiences and exposures. Documentation in official records (e.g., law enforcement records, medical charts) also needs to be improved so that more research can be conducted using available records. An improvement in official records would reduce, to some degree, the need for and expense associated with investigating certain research questions in one-time studies.

Recommendation: National and community level representative sample survey studies using the most valid instrumentation and questioning techniques available to measure incidence and prevalence of violence against

women are needed. These studies should collect data not only on behavior, but also on injuries and other consequences of violence. Studies of incidence and prevalence of perpetration of violence against women are also needed. National and community surveys of other topics, such as women's mental or physical health or social or economic well being, should be encouraged to include questions pertaining to violence against women. Furthermore, identification and secondary analysis of existing data sets with respect to violence against women should be funded.

Research on Context

A consideration of the context in which women experience violence is vital to understanding the nature of the problem, as well as to the consequences to the woman, and effectiveness of interventions. There is little understanding of how such factors as race, ethnicity, socioeconomic status, culture, and sexual orientation intersect with gender to shape the particular context in which violence occurs. Because women's experiences differ on these dimensions, those differences must be understood and incorporated into the body of knowledge about violence against women in order to design intervention strategies. Other factors that warrant consideration include disability, religion, homelessness, and institutionalization. Investigators should be encouraged to undertake studies that examine risk factors for victimization as well as groups at risk of victimization. In other words, in addition to identifying target groups for prevention and intervention, research needs to identify elements that might be amenable to change.

Recommendation: All research on violence against women should take into account the context within which women live their lives and in which the violence occurs. This context should include the broad social and cultural context, as well as individual factors. Work should in-

clude more qualitative research, such as ethnographic research, as well as quantitative research, designed to uncover the confluence of factors such as race, socioeconomic status, age, and sexual orientation in shaping the context and experience of violence in women's lives.

NOTES

1. The UCR does not provide data on homicides for Hispanic or Asian Americans.

2. The National Crime Victimization Survey has been well described and its limitations examined in other work; see, for example, Reiss and Roth (1993), Fagan and Browne (1994), and Koss (1992, 1993).

3. The terms "Hispanic" and "Latino/Latina" are used interchangeably in this report, following the term used in the research being reported.

4. For a detailed discussion of the validity and reliability of the Conflict Tactics Scales, see Straus (1990b,c).

3
Causes and Consequences of Violence Against Women

CAUSES

A vital part of understanding a social problem, and a precursor to preventing it, is an understanding of what causes it. Research on the causes of violence against women has consisted of two lines of inquiry: examination of the characteristics that influence the behavior of offenders and consideration of whether some women have a heightened vulnerability to victimization. Research has sought causal factors at various levels of analysis, including individual, dyadic, institutional, and social. Studies of offending and victimization remain conceptually distinct except in sociocultural analysis in which joint consideration is often given to two complementary processes: those that influence men to be aggressive and channel their expressions of violence toward women and those that position women for receipt of violence and operate to silence them afterwards. Many theorists and researchers have sought to answer the question, "Why does this particular man batter or sexually assault?" by looking at single classes of influences. Among them have been biologic factors such as androgenic hormonal influences; evolutionary theories; intrapsychic explanations focused on mental disorder or personality traits and profiles; social learning models that highlight the socialization experiences that shape individual men to be violent; social information processing theory concerning the cognitive processes that offenders engage in before, during, and after violence; sociocultural analyses aimed at understanding the structural features of society at the level of the dyad, family, peer group, school, religion, media, and state that encourage male violence and maintain women as a vulnerable class of potential victims; and feminist explanations stressing the gendered nature of violence against women and its roots in patriarchal social systems. Recently, researchers armed with multivariate statistical analysis have tested complex models of violence with multiple factors to explain battering (McKenry et al., 1995) and to model the common roots of verbal, physical, and sexual coercion toward women (Malamuth et al., 1995). Also new are integrative metatheories of intimate violence that consider the impact of historical, sociocultural, and social factors on people, including the processes whereby social influences are transmitted to and represented within individual psychological functioning, including cognition and motivation (White, in press).

Many of the theories about the causes of perpetrating violence against women are drawn from the literature on aggression and general violence. Both the research on general violence and that on violence against women suggest that violence arises from interactions among individual biological and psychosocial factors and social processes (e.g., Reiss and Roth, 1993), but it is not known how much overlap there is in the development of violent behavior against women and other violent behavior. Studies of male batterers have found that some batterers confine their violent behavior to their intimates but others are violent in general (Fagan et al., 1983; Cadsky and Crawford, 1988; Shields et al., 1988; Saunders, 1992; Holtzworth-Munroe and Stuart, 1994). The research suggests that, at least in some cases, there may be differences in the factors that cause violence against women and those that cause other violent behavior. Much more work is needed in order to understand in what ways violence against women differs from other violent behavior. Such understanding will be particularly important for developing preventive interventions.

Although current understanding suggests that violent behavior is not caused by any single factor, much of the research has focused on single causes. Therefore, in the following sections several salient findings emerging from each single-factor domain are highlighted to illustrate how each contributes something to the causal nexus of perpetration of violence. They are followed by a brief review of efforts to build multifactor models.

Theories of Violent Offending

Individual Determinants

Evolution From an evolutionary perspective, the goal of sexual behavior is to maximize the likelihood of passing on one's genes. This goal involves maximizing the chances that one will have offspring who themselves will survive to reproduce. In ancestral environments, optimum male and female strategies for successfully passing on one's genes often did not coincide because the amount of parental investment required by males is smaller than that required by females. Males were best served by mating with as many fertile females as possible to increase their chance of impregnating one of them; females, who have the tasks of pregnancy and nurturing the young, are often better served by pair bonding. Sex differences in current human mating strategies may be explained as having been shaped by the strategies that created reproductive success among human ancestors. A number of studies have shown that young adult males are more interested in partner variety, less interested in committed long-term relationships, and more willing to engage in impersonal sex than are young adult females (Clark and Hatfield, 1989; Symons and Ellis, 1989; Clark, 1990; Landolt et al., 1995). This finding is consistent with the optimum evolutionary strategy for males of mating with as many fertile females as possible.

It is theorized that males who have difficulty obtaining partners are more likely to resort to sexual coercion or rape. Extensive evidence of forced mating among animals has been documented (Ellis, 1989). Evolutionary theory also has been used to explain aspects of intimate partner violence. It is theorized that male sexual jealousy developed as a means of assuring the paternity of their offspring (Quinsey and Lalumière, 1995). Case histories from battered women often mention the extreme sexual jealousy displayed by their batterers (Walker, 1979; Browne, 1987), and extreme sexual jealousy is a common motive of men who kill their wives (Daly and Wilson, 1988).

There is much debate over how much influence evolutionary factors have on modern human beings. Even those who favor evolutionary explanations acknowledge that additional factors are necessary to explain sexual assault and intimate partner violence. For example, Quinsey and Lalumière (1995) suggest that rape and other sexual coercion may be explained by the evolutionary approach that is modified by specific attitudes toward women or by psychopathy, coupled with an erotic interest in coercive sexual behavior. Evolutionary explanations of rape are also criticized as not explaining the proportion of rapes lacking reproductive consequences because they involve oral or anal penetration or victims who are prepubescent or male.

Physiology and Neurophysiology The physiological or neurophysiological correlates of violence and aggression that have received particular attention are the functioning of steroid hormones such as testosterone; the functioning of neurotransmitters such as serotonin, dopamine, norepinephrine, acetylcholine, and gamma-aminobutyric acid (GABA); neuroanatomical abnormalities; neurophysiological abnormalities; and brain dysfunctions that interfere with cognition or language processing. This literature has been well reviewed in other sources (e.g., Fishbein, 1990; Reiss and Roth, 1993; Brain, 1994; Miczek et al., 1994a,b; Mirsky and Siegel, 1994); this section highlights the overall findings and notes studies that have specifically looked at violence against women. In considering this literature, it should be remembered that much of the evidence comes from animal studies and that generalizing from animals to humans is not straightforward. The evidence that comes from studies of human subjects only shows correlations, so any causal interpretations are tenuous. Furthermore, changes in hormonal, neurotransmitter, and neurophysiological processes may be consequences of violent behavior or victimization, as well as being causes of those behaviors (Reiss and Roth, 1993; van der Kolk, 1994).

A recent comprehensive literature review (Archer, 1991) concluded that the majority of studies showed that high testosterone levels tend to covary with high probabilities of aggressive behaviors, dominance status, and pathological forms of aggression in nonhuman mammals, but that the picture for humans is not as clear. In humans, there appears to be a correlation between testosterone levels and aggression, but it is not clear whether testosterone levels influence aggressive behavior or vary as a result of aggressive behavior. Similarly, the results of human studies of neurotransmitters are not conclusive. For example, low levels of serotonin, the most heavily studied of the neurotransmitters, have been found to be correlated with aggressive behavior, impulsivity, and suicidal behavior (Asberg et al., 1976; Brown et al., 1979; Linnoila et al., 1983; Lidberg et al., 1985; Mann, 1987; Coccaro et al., 1989). More recent studies have found a complex interaction among serotonin, alcoholism, and monoamine metabolism and these behaviors (Linnoila et al., 1989; Virkkunen et al., 1989a,b). Further evidence of the role of neurotransmitters comes from the fact that drugs that act on serotonin receptors or on monoamine oxidase may reduce aggressiveness. Animal and human studies have found trauma and violence to have effects on hormones, neurotransmitters, and brain function (e.g., van der Kolk, 1994).

Studies have also looked at brain abnormalities and violent behavior. Neuropsychological deficits in memory, attention, and language, which sometimes follow limbic system damage, have been found to be common in children who exhibit violent or aggressive behavior (e.g., Miller, 1987; Lewis et al., 1988; Mungas, 1988). Differences in peripheral measures of nervous system activity, such as heart rate or skin conductance, have been found between control subjects and samples of criminals, psychopaths, delinquents, and conduct-disordered children (Siddle et al., 1973; Wadsworth, 1976; Raine and Venables, 1988; Kagan, 1989; Raine et al., 1990). Langevin (1990:112) found a "link between temporal lobe impairment and sexually anomalous behaviors" that was independent of nonsexual criminality and not explained by learning disabilities or alcohol abuse. Reduced impulse control and personality changes following head injury may lead to an increased risk of battering (Detre et al., 1975; Lewis et al., 1986, 1988). Likewise, studies have found that batterers are more likely to have had head injuries than nonbatterers (Rosenbaum and Hoge, 1989; Rosenbaum et al., 1996).

There is increasing interest in the role played by biological factors in violent behavior; however, most researchers believe it is the interaction of biological, developmental, and environmental factors that is important (Fishbein, 1990). For example, Marshall and Barbaree (1990) speculate that biological factors may set the stage for learning, providing limits and possibilities rather than determining outcomes, and that developmental and environmental factors play the larger role. However, as suggested by a previous study (Reiss and Roth, 1993), preventing head injuries and environmental exposure to toxins, such as lead, that may damage brain functioning could be considered potential avenues for preventing violence.

Alcohol Every category of aggressive act (except throwing objects) has a higher prevalence among people who have been drinking (Pernanen, 1976). Alcohol use has been reported in between 25 percent and 85 percent of incidents of battering and up to 75 percent of acquaintance rapes (Kantor and Straus, 1987; Muehlenhard and Linton, 1987; Koss et al., 1988). It is far more prevalent for men than their female victims. Considerable research links drinking and alcohol abuse to physical aggression, although adult consumption patterns are likewise associated with other variables related to violence (such as witnessing physical violence in one's home of origin; Kantor, 1993). The relationship of alcohol to intimate partner violence could be spurious, but the relationship of men's drinking to intimate partner violence remains even after statistically controlling for sociodemographic variables, hostility, and marital satisfaction (Leonard and Blane, 1992; Leonard, 1993). Men's drinking patterns, especially binge drinking, are associated with marital violence across all ethnic groups and social classes (Kantor, 1993).

The relationship of alcohol to violence is a complex one, involving physiological, psychosocial, and sociocultural factors. The exact effects of alcohol on the central nervous system remain in question, but nonexperimental evidence indicates that alcohol may interact with neurotransmitters, such as serotonin, that have been associated with effects on aggression (Linnoila et al., 1983; Virkkunen et al., 1989a,b). Studies have found a genetic basis for alcohol abuse and alcoholism (Cloninger et al., 1978; Plomin, 1989) and for antisocial personality traits (Christiansen, 1977; Bohman et al., 1982; Mednick et al., 1984; Cloninger and Gottesman, 1987) that are often found among violent offenders. The fact that alcohol abuse and antisocial personality frequently occur together has led to the speculation of common genetic bases, but the evidence remains inconclusive (Reiss and Roth, 1993).

Alcohol may interfere with cognitive processes, in particular, social cognitions. Recent studies suggest that men under the influence of alcohol are more likely to misperceive ambiguous or neutral cues as suggestive of sexual interest and to ignore or misinterpret cues that a woman is unwilling

(Abbey et al., 1995). The impact of alcohol on behavior has also been linked to a person's expectations about alcohol's effects. For example, Lang et al. (1975) found individuals became more aggressive in laboratory experiments after drinking what they were told was alcohol, even though it was not. Similarly, laboratory studies of penile responses to pornographic stimuli decrease with actual ingestion of alcohol, but increase when participants believe they have drunk alcohol when they have actually received a placebo drink (Richardson and Hammock, 1991). It has also been suggested that alcohol may be used to excuse violent behavior (Coleman and Straus, 1983; Collins, 1986). These deviance disavowal theories ("I wouldn't have done it if I hadn't been drunk") have not been empirically tested, however (Kantor, 1993).

There are methodological weaknesses in the studies of the links between alcohol and violence, including lack of clear definitions of excessive alcohol use and a reliance on clinical samples with an absence of control samples. (For a more complete review of the research and methodological weaknesses see Leonard and Jacob, 1988; Leonard, 1993.) Nonetheless, research has consistently found that heavy drinking patterns are related to aggressive behavior, in general, and to intimate partner and sexual violence. However, exactly how alcohol is related to violence remains unclear. Obviously, many battering incidents and sexual assaults occur in the absence of alcohol, and many people drink without engaging in violent behavior (Kantor and Straus, 1990).

Psychopathology and Personality Traits   A number of studies have found a high incidence of psychopathology and personality disorders, most frequently antisocial personality disorder, borderline personality organization, or posttraumatic stress syndrome, among men who assault their wives (Hamberger and Hastings, 1986, 1988, 1991; Hart et al., 1993; Dutton and Starzomski, 1993; Dutton, 1994, 1995; Dutton et al., 1994). A wide variety of psychiatric and personality disorders have also been diagnosed among sexual offenders, most frequently some type of antisocial personality disorder (Prentky, 1990).

Distinctive personality profiles have been reported for rapists and sexually aggressive men (Groth and Birnbaum, 1979; Abel et al., 1986), and batterers (Geffner and Rosenbaum, 1990). However, personality testing of rapists has found no significant differences between sexual offenders and those incarcerated for nonsexual offenses (Quinsey et al., 1980; Langevin, 1983). Studies of the personalities of incarcerated rapists and court-referred batterers are problematic; these men are typically poorly educated and from low-status occupations. Thus the differences may say more about who gets reported, arrested, tried, convicted, and sentenced than it does about the personalities of violent men. Rape, for example, is one of the most underreported crimes (Bowker, 1979), and only a small proportion of reported rapes result in incarceration (Darke, 1990). Even within the restricted population found in studies of incarcerated sex offenders, most investigators have concluded that there is a great deal of heterogeneity among rapists and that sexual aggression is multiply determined (Prentky and Knight, 1991).

Batterers also seem to be a heterogeneous group (Gondolf, 1988; Saunders, 1992). Because of this heterogeneity, much of the research on incarcerated rapists and known batterers has included attempts to develop typologies to represent subgroups of them. Typologies of batterers have generally used one, or a combination, of three dimensions to distinguish between subgroups: frequency and severity of physical violence and related sexual or psychological abuse; generality of the violence (i.e., violence only in the family or violence in general); and psychopathology or personality disorder (Holtzworth-Munroe and Stuart, 1994). Rapists have been categorized by motivational factors (sexual or aggressive), impulse control factors, and social competence. (For a detailed description of sexual offender taxonomies, see Knight and Prentky, 1990.)

Because incarcerated sexual offenders and batterers in treatment are probably not representative of all sex offenders or batterers, another avenue of research has focused on normal population samples, comparing those who self-report physically or sexually aggressive behavior and those who do not. Sexually aggressive men are said to differ from other men in antisocial tendencies (Malamuth, 1986), nonconformity (Rapaport and Burkhart, 1984), impulsivity (Calhoun, 1990), and hypermasculinity (Mosher and Anderson, 1986). Batterers have been found to show lower socialization and responsibility (Barnett and Hamberger, 1992). It is important to remember, however, that there are potential biases in self-report data, and it is difficult to verify their accuracy other than through consistency of responses. Men may be reluctant to acknowledge that they have engaged in sexually or physically violent behavior or the men who report this behavior may be different from those who have engaged in the behavior but do not report it. Yet, because both intimate partner violence and sexual assault usually take place in private, self-reports play a central role in their study. Self-report measures on sensitive topics, including violent behaviors, have been found to be quite reliable (Straus, 1979; Hindelang et al., 1981; Bridges and Weis, 1989).

Attitudes and Gender Schemas   Cultural myths about violence, gender scripts and roles, sexual scripts and roles, and male entitlements are represented at the individual level as attitudes and gender schemas. These hypothetical entities are expectancies that give meaning to and may even bias interpretation of ongoing experience, as well as provide a structure for the range of possible responses. Acceptance of beliefs that have been shown to foster rape has been demonstrated among a variety of Americans, including typical citizens, police officers, and judges (Field, 1978; Burt, 1980; Mahoney et al., 1986). Once a violence-supportive schema about women has developed, men are more likely to misinterpret ambiguous evidence as confirming their beliefs (Abbey, 1991). Sexually aggressive men more strongly endorse a set of attitudes that are supportive of rape than do nonaggressive men, including myths about rape and the use of interpersonal violence as a strategy for resolving conflict (e.g., Malamuth, 1986; Malamuth et al., 1991, 1995). Beliefs and myths about rape may serve as rationalizations for those who commit violent acts. For example, incarcerated rapists often rationalize that their victim either desired or deserved to experience forced sexual acts. Similarly, culturally sanctioned beliefs about the rights and privileges of husbands have historically legitimized a man's domination over his wife and warranted his use of violence to control her. Men, in general, are more accepting of men abusing women, and the most culturally traditional men are the most accepting (Greenblatt, 1985). Batterers' often excuse their violence by pointing to their wives' "unwifely" behavior as their justification (Dobash and Dobash, 1979; Adams, 1988; Ptacek, 1988).

Sex and Power Motives   Violence against women is widely believed to be motivated by needs to dominate women. This view conjures the image of a powerful man who uses violence against women as a tool to maintain his superiority, but research suggests that the relationship is more complex. Power and control frequently underlie intimate partner violence, but the purpose of the violence may also be in response to a man's feelings of powerlessness and inability to accept rejection (Browne and Dutton, 1990). It also has been argued that rape, in particular, represents fulfillment of sexual needs through violence (Ellis, 1989), but research has found that motives of power and anger are more prominent in the rationalizations for sexual aggression than sexual desires (Lisak and Roth, 1990; Lisak, 1994). Attempts to resolve the debate about sex versus power have involved laboratory studies of men's sexual arousal to stimuli of depictions of pure violence, pure consensual sex, and nonconsensual sex plus violence. These studies have consistently shown that some "normal" males with no known history of rape may be aroused by rape stimuli involving adult women, especially if the women are portrayed as enjoying the experience (Hall, 1990). However, sexually aggressive men appear to be more sexually arousable in general, either to consenting or rape stimuli (Rapaport and Posey, 1991), and rapists respond more than nonsexual offenders to rape cues than to consenting sex cues (Lalumière and Quinsey, 1994). Sexually aggressive men openly admit that their sexual fantasies are dominated by aggressive and sadistic material (Greendlinger and Byrne, 1987; Quinsey, 1984).

Social Learning   Social learning theory posits that humans learn social behavior by observing others' behavior and the consequences of that behavior, forming ideas about what behaviors are appropriate, trying those behaviors, and continuing them if the results are positive (O'Leary, 1988). This theory does not view aggression as inevitable, but rather sees it as a social behavior that is learned and shaped by its consequences, continuing if it is reinforced (Lore and Schultz, 1993). From this perspective, male violence against women endures in human societies because it is modeled both in individual families and in the society more generally and has positive results: it releases tension, leaves the perpetrator feeling better, often achieves its ends by cutting off arguments, and is rarely associated with serious punishment for the perpetrator.

One of the mechanisms through which social learning occurs is social information processing—the decoding or interpreting of social interactions, making decisions about appropriate responses on the basis of the decoding, and carrying out a response to see if it has the intended effect. It has been hypothesized that violent men may be deficient in the skills necessary to accurately decode communications from women. For example, men's judgments of videotapes of male-female interactions are more highly sexualized than women's judgments (Abbey, 1991; Kowalski, 1992, 1993). Batterers appear to be more likely than nonviolent men to attribute negative intentions to their partners' actions and to behave negatively, for example, with anger or contempt (Dutton and Browning, 1988; Margolin et al., 1988; Holtzworth-Munroe, 1992).

Dyadic Contexts

An individual man carries out violence against a woman in a dyadic context that includes features of the relationship, characteristics of the woman, and their communication. The stage of relationship between a man and woman may determine, in part, the probability of violence. Anecdotal evidence from battered women suggest that a man often refrains from physical violence until a women has made an emotional commitment to him, such as moving in together, getting engaged or married, or becoming pregnant (e.g., Walker, 1979; Giles-Sims, 1983; Browne, 1987). It is suggested that the emotional bond between the couple once formed, may contribute to the man's sense of entitlement to control his partner's behavior as well as diminish the facility with which the woman can leave the relationship without ambivalence. Some evidence suggests that women are willing to see the first violent incident as an anomaly, and so are willing to forgive it, although this response may actually reinforce the violent behavior (Giles-Sims, 1983).

Acquaintance or date rape may also be related to relationship stage, with different risk factors for rapes during first dates and rapes in on-going relationships (Shotland, 1992). For example, men who rape on first or second dates may be similar to stranger rapists, while men who rape early in a developing relationship may misperceive their partners' intent (Shotland, 1992). Prior sexual intimacy between partners may increase a man's belief that he has a right to such intimacy any time he desires it, and it may also support his false assumption that a forced sexual encounter in an experienced woman is harmless (Johnson and Jackson, 1988). Completed rapes have been found to be more likely in couples who know each other well than among persons who are acquaintances (Belnap, 1989). As noted in the section on social learning (above), physically and sexually aggressive men may misinterpret cues from females. It has been found, for example, that male batterers have poor communication skills (Ganley and Harris, 1978; Holtzworth-Monroe and Anglin, 1991).

Institutional Influences

Family, Schools, and Religion   Families are where all socialization begins, including socialization for all types of violent behavior. Studies of violent criminals and violent sex offenders have found these men are more likely than other adults to have experienced poor parental childrearing, poor supervision, physical abuse, neglect, and separations from their parents (Langevin et al., 1985; Farrington, 1991). Increased risk of adult intimate partner violence is associated with exposure to violence between a person's parents while growing up. One-third of children who have been abused or exposed to parental violence become violent adults (Widom, 1989). Sons of violent parents are more likely to abuse their intimate partners than boys from nonviolent homes (Straus et al., 1980). Men raised in patriarchal family structures in which traditional gender roles are encouraged are more likely to become violent adults, to rape women acquaintances, and to batter their intimate partners than men raised in more egalitarian homes (Straus et al., 1980; Gwartney-Gibbs et al., 1983; Fagot et al., 1988; Friedrich et al., 1988; Koss and Dinero, 1989; Riggs and O'Leary, 1989; Malamuth et al., 1991, 1995). Sexual abuse in childhood has been identified as a risk factor in males for sexual offending as an adult (Groth and Birnbaum, 1979; Briere, 1992). Experiences of sexual abuse in one's family may lead to inaccurate notions about healthy sexuality, inappropriate justifications for violent behavior, failure to develop personal boundaries, and contribute to communication and coping styles that rely on denial, reinterpretation of experiences, and avoidance (Briere, 1992; Herman, 1992).

To the extent that schools reinforce sex role stereotypes and attitudes that condone the use of violence, they may contribute to socialization supportive of violent behavior. Other institutions that have been implicated in contributing to socialization that supports violence against women are organized religion (Fortune, 1983; Whipple, 1987), the workplace (Fitzgerald, 1993), the U.S. military (Russell, 1989), and the media (Linz et al., 1992).

Athletic teams also may socialize children to behavior that is supportive of violence. For example, male athletes may be spurred to greater aggressive efforts by coaches who deride them as "girls." Participation in revenue-producing sports at the collegiate level was found to be a significant predictor of sexual aggression among college students (Koss and Gaines, 1993). It is possible that team sports, particularly revenue-producing sports, attract young men who are already aggressive. Whether team sports encourage aggressive behavior or simply reinforce already existing aggressive tendencies remains to be determined. In either case, it appears that participation in team sports is a risk factor for sexual aggression.

Media Many feminist writers (e.g., Brownmiller, 1975; Dworkin, 1991; Russell, 1993) have suggested that pornography encourages the objectification of women and endorses and condones sexual aggression toward women. Both laboratory research and studies of television lend support to this view. Exposure to pornography under laboratory conditions has been found to increase men's aggression toward women, particularly when a male participant has been affronted, insulted, or provoked by a woman (Linz et al., 1992). Sexual arousal to depictions of rape is characteristic of sexual offenders (Hall, 1990). Even exposure to nonexplicit sexual scenes with graphic violence has been shown to decrease empathy for rape victims (Linz et al., 1988). It appears that it is the depiction of violence against women more than sexual explicitness that results in callousness toward female victims of violence and attitudes that are accepting of such violence (Donnerstein and Linz, 1994).

It is not only pornography that depicts violence against women. Television and movies are filled with scenes of women being threatened, raped, beaten, tortured, and murdered. A number of studies of television point to the deleterious effects of viewing media portrayals of violence (e.g., Eron, 1982; National Institute of Mental Health, 1982; Huston et al., 1992). Eron (1982) found that children who watched many hours of violence on television during elementary school tended to exhibit more aggressive behavior as teenagers and were more likely to be arrested for criminal acts as adults. A meta-analysis of 188 studies found a strong positive association between exposure to television violence and antisocial and aggressive behavior (Comstock and Paik, 1990; Paik and Comstock, 1994). Those who are exposed to television and cinema violence may also become desensitized to real world violence, less sensitive to the pain and suffering of others, and begin to see the world as a mean and dangerous place (Murray, 1995). A recently released national study of violence on television found that context of the violence shown was important: television shows virtually no consequences of violent behavior; victims are not harmed and offenders are not punished (Mediascope, 1996). It seems that many television depictions of violence send the message that violence works.

None of the studies of television violence has focused specifically on violence against women. The National Television Violence Study (Mediascope, 1996) found that 75 percent of the targets of violence in television portrayals are males, while only 9 percent are females (the remainder are nonhuman characters). Research has not yet examined the type of violence directed at female victims on television, how it compares with that directed at male victims, and whether there are differential effects on viewers of violence against women and against men.

Societal Influences

For much of recorded Western European and American

history, wives had no independent legal status; they were basically their husbands' property. The right of a husband to physically chastise his wife was upheld by the Supreme Court of Mississippi in 1824 (*Bradley v. State*, 1 Miss. 157) and again by a court in North Carolina in 1868 (*State v. Rhodes*, 61 N.C. 453, 353; cited in Pleck, 1989). In 1871 a court ruling in Alabama (*Fulgham v. State*, 46 Ala. 146-147) made that state the first to rescind a husband's right to beat his wife (Fagan and Browne, 1994). During the 1870s, coinciding with the rise of the child protective movement, there was increased concern that wife beating should be treated as a crime, although few men were ever punished (Pleck, 1989). In the 1890s social casework replaced criminal justice as the preferred system for dealing with family violence and general interest in wife beating waned until the 1960s (Fagan and Browne, 1994).

The status of women as property also can be seen in the development of laws concerning rape. Brownmiller (1975:8) contends that "rape entered the law . . . as a property crime of man against man. Woman, of course, was viewed as the property." She notes that until the end of the thirteenth century, only unmarried virgins were considered blameless in their victimization; married women who were raped were punished along with their rapist. At that time, the Statutes of Westminister put forward by Edward I of England extended the same penalties to men who raped married women as to those who raped virgins. Rape within marriage, however, was, by definition, impossible. Marriage laws traditionally assumed implied consent to sexual relations by wives and allowed husbands to use force to gain compliance (Fagan and Browne, 1994). It has only been in recent years that laws have begun to recognize marital rape: today every state in the United States has modified or eliminated the marriage exclusion in its rape laws (personal communication, National Clearinghouse on Marital and Date Rape, Berkeley, California).

Sexual Scripts   Expectations about dating and intimate relationships are conveyed by culturally transmitted scripts. Scripts support violence when they encourage men to feel superior, entitled, and licensed as sexual aggressors with women as their prey, while holding women responsible for controlling the extent of sexual involvement (White and Koss, 1993). Parents socialize daughters to resist sexual advances and sons to initiate sexual activity (Ross, 1977). By adolescence, both boys and girls have been found to endorse scripts about sexual interaction that delineate a justifiable rape. For example, approximately 25 percent of middle school, high school, and college students state that it is acceptable for a man to force sex on a woman if he spent money on her (Goodchilds and Zellman, 1984; Muehlenhard et al., 1985; Goodchilds et al., 1988).

Since Burt (1980) first defined "rape myths" and developed a scale to measure them, a large body of research has examined the role of attitudes and false beliefs about rape on perpetration of sexual assault and on society's response to sexual assault. Typical rape myths include denial of rape's existence (e.g., most rape claims are false, or women generally lie about rape), excusing the rape (e.g., she led him on, he couldn't help himself, rape only happens to "bad" women), and minimizing the seriousness of rape (e.g., Hall et al., 1986; Briere et al., 1985). Despite psychometrically weak measurement instruments, the study of rape myths has provided important understandings about sexual aggression (Lonsway and Fitzgerald, 1994). Not surprisingly, men are more accepting of rape myths than women (e.g., Muehlenhard and Linton, 1987; Margolin et al., 1989; Dye and Roth, 1990). A number of studies have found a significant association between acceptance of rape myths and self-reported sexually aggressive behavior (Field 1978; Koss et al., 1985; Murphy et al., 1986; Muehlenhard and Linton, 1987; Reilly et al., 1992).

The early studies of rape myths were performed on college campuses and found that 25 percent to 35 percent of the students accepted a variety of them (Giacopassi and Dull, 1986; Gilmartin-Zena, 1987). Since the mid 1980s, many college campuses have instituted rape awareness and rape education programs. Recent research found fewer than 2 percent of students accepting of sexual aggression or coercion, but up to 36 percent expected that sexual aggression would occur under certain circumstances (Cook, 1995). Cook (1995) surmises that rape education has made it unacceptable to admit to believing rape myths, but that behavioral expectations are still consistent with acceptance of rape myths. It will be valuable for prevention efforts for research to continue to track any changes in rape myth acceptance and sexual script expectations among students, as well as the general public.

Cultural Mores   Ethnographic and anthropologic studies determine the critical role that sociocultural mores play in defining and promoting violence against women. Anthropologists have found cultural differences in the amount of and acceptability of intimate partner violence in different societies. A review of 14 different societies (Counts et al., 1992) found that physical chastisement of wives was tolerated in all the societies and considered necessary in many societies, but the rates and severity of wife beating were found to range from almost nonexistent to very frequent. These differences seem to be related to negative sanctions for men who overstepped "acceptable" limits, sanctuaries for women to escape violence, and a sense of honor based on nonviolence or decent treatment of women (Campbell, 1992).

Two general types of rape have been identified. Transgressive or non-normative rape is uncondoned genital contact against the will of the woman and in violation of social norms; tolerated or normative rape is unwanted genital contact that is supported by social norms (Heise, 1993; Rozee, 1993). Normative rape is reported in nearly all societies (97 percent; Rozee, 1993), and all have mechanisms that "legitimate, obfuscate, deny, and thereby perpetuate violence" (Heise et al., 1994:1). Ethnographic studies have found rape in 42 percent to 90 percent of nonindustrial societies, depending on how it is defined and on the cultural and geographic representativeness of the sample (Minturn et al., 1969; Bart et al., 1975; Broude and Green, 1976; Sanday, 1981; Levinson, 1989; Rozee, 1993; for a review see Koss et al., 1994). In preliterate societies, there were significantly greater frequencies of rape in those characterized by patrilocality, high degree of interpersonal violence, and an ideology of male toughness. Rape is also prevalent under conditions of marked social inequity and social disorganization, such as slavery and war (Quinsey, 1984).

Multifactor Models

It is generally accepted that multiple classes of influences—from the individual to the macrolevel—determine the expression of assaultive and sexually aggressive behavior in men (for recent reviews see Ellis, 1989; Sugarman and Hotaling, 1989; Craig, 1990; Hall, 1990; Malamuth and Dean, 1991; Berkowitz, 1992; Shotland, 1992; White and Koss, 1993; White, in press). Although it is possible to model at a general level the causal factors that explain the variance among the forms of violence against women, the heterogeneity of violent men precludes the delineation of a single set of causes that accurately classifies types of offenders. Therefore, researchers have turned to multivariate modeling of violence. Recent efforts include a biopsychosocial model of battering that examines the relative contribution of three domains of predictors including the physical (e.g., testosterone, prolactin, and alcohol), the social (e.g., negative life events, quality of relationships, family income, and social support), and psychiatric symptoms (McKenry et al., 1995). The results showed significant zero-order correlations within each class of predictors, but in multivariate analysis the social variables predicted violence better than the other variables.

Work by Malamuth and colleagues (1991, 1993, 1995) has generated and tested a model to explain both sexual and nonsexual aggression toward women. Their results suggest that there are common pathways to all forms of aggression, but different specific factors may influence the development of nonsexual versus sexual aggression toward women. Furthermore, some of the same factors that contribute to sexual aggression in early adulthood appear to lead to other conflictual behaviors with women in later life. Male sexual aggression was best predicted by a history of promiscuous-impersonal sex and distrust of women coupled with gratification from dominating them. Physical aggression was best predicted by relationship distress and verbal aggression. General hostility and defensiveness contributed to both types of aggression. This work supports the findings of other researchers (O'Leary and Arias, 1988; O'Leary et al., 1994) that psychological abuse may be a precursor to physical aggression. These findings point to the need for more work that looks at commonalities and differences among all forms of violence against women and general violence.

All this work is a marked improvement over earlier research that focused on single causes or theories. The field appears to be developing toward an integrative, metatheoretical model of violence that considers multiple variables operating at different times in a probabilistic fashion (Leonard, 1993; White, in press). Future work guided by these models can examine the relationship of one form of violence to another; make better connections between macrolevel societal variables and individual variables to establish how culture is expressed; address both structural and contextual causes of violence; use a life-span perspective capable of capturing the processes by which earlier experiences affect later ones; and focus on the gendered nature of violence against women that involves personality and cognitive factors embedded in a social structure that directs and defines the meaning of violence in gendered social relationships. An understanding of the multiple factors that lead to violent behavior in general and to specific forms of violent behavior directed at women is critical to developing effective prevention strategies.

Risk Factors for Victimization

Although most research on the causes of violence focuses on why men use violence and the conditions that support and maintain that violence, some researchers have tried to ask why a particular woman is the target of violence. This line of research has a dismal record of success. A primary problem confronted in trying to identify women's risk factors for violence is the confounding that occurs when traits and behaviors are assessed at some point postvictimization and assumed to represent the previctimization state. An interpretation of current findings is that they represent aftereffects of the violence itself or overly negative self-descriptions triggered by the trauma.

Factors that have been at one time or another linked to women's likelihood of being raped or battered are passivity, hostility, low self-esteem, alcohol and drug use, violence in the family of origin, having more education or income than their intimate partners, and the use of violence toward children. However, based on a critical review of all 52 studies conducted in the prior 15 years that included comparison groups, Hotaling and Sugarman (1986) found that the only risk marker consistently associated with being the victim of physical abuse was having witnessed parental violence as a child. And this factor characterized not only the victimized women, but also their male assailants. Recent studies also found no specific personality and attitudinal characteristics that make certain women more vulnerable to battering (e.g., Pittman and Taylor, 1992). Although alcoholic women are more likely to report moderate to severe violence in their relationships than more moderate drinkers, the association disappears after controlling for alcohol problems in their partners (Miller, 1992, as cited in Leonard, 1993). On the basis of findings such as these, several writers have concluded that the major risk factor for battering is being a woman.

Personality traits and attitudes that could increase vulnerability to rape have also been explored. The earliest studies, and the only ones to implicate victim personality traits, used different recruitment techniques to obtain subjects: the rape victims were often found among those who had sought help at crisis centers; the nonvictims were college student volunteers (Selkin, 1978; Myers et al., 1984). These methodological differences bias the samples, especially on personality traits like dominance, femininity, and social presence—exactly the variables on which the groups were found to differ. When identical selection procedures were used to select victims and nonvictims, no differences were found in personality characteristics, assertiveness, or identification with feminine stereotyped behavior (Koss, 1985; Koss and Dinero, 1989).

One risk profile did emerge that characterized a small subset (10 percent) of women for whom the risk of rape was twice the rate for women without the profile. Those women were characterized by a background of childhood sexual abuse, liberal sexual attitudes, and higher than average alcohol use and larger number of sexual partners. Researchers presume that having a large number of sexual partners implies short-term relationships and therefore more dating partners, but neither frequency of dates nor number of dating partners has been directly tested as a risk factor. Koss and Dinero (1989) concluded that sexual assault was generally not predictable, but to the extent it could be, was accounted for by variables that represented the aftereffects of childhood sexual abuse, including influences on drinking, sexual values, and level of sexual activity. Recent prospective data support this assertion (Gidycz et al., 1995). Adolescent sexual victimization significantly predicted alcohol consumption at the onset of college, while alcohol consumption during college did not predict subsequent victimization. The link between childhood sexual abuse and adult victimization has been replicated many times across ethnic groups (Wyatt et al., 1992; Gidycz et al., 1993; Urquiza and Goodlin-Jones, 1994; Wyatt and Riederle, 1994). The other certain risk factor for rape (in addition to being female and having been abused previously) is being young: epidemiological data indicate that women between 16 and 24 years old have the highest rates of sexual assault and rape (Bastian, 1995).

Another line of research has compared the resistance strategies used by women who were raped to those of women whose attack was aborted without penetration. Studies of this type have consistently reported that active strategies such as screaming, fleeing, or physically struggling are associated with higher rates of rape avoidance (Javorek, 1979; Bart, 1981; Quinsey and Upfold, 1985; Levine-MacCombie and Koss, 1986; Siegel et al., 1989; Ullman and Knight, 1991, 1992). Although some of the studies found increased risk of injury among women who resisted, the studies that looked at the actual sequence of events (Quinsey and Upfold, 1985; Ullman and Knight, 1992) found the correlation between resistance and injury disappeared when the violence of the attacker was taken into account. Researchers have uniformly found that offender characteristics are more important than the victim behavior in predicting the outcome of an assault.

The role of alcohol use by victims has also been investigated. Trouble with alcohol and peer pressure to drink have been associated with adolescents' risks of personal victimization, in general, and sexual victimization, in particular (Esbensen and Huizinga, 1991; Windle, 1994; Gidycz et al., 1995). About one-half of college student rape victims report that they were drinking at the time of their assault (Koss and Dinero, 1989), and estimated peak blood alcohol level during the prior 30 days was correlated with lifetime sexual victimization (Norris et al., 1996). Alcohol use is one of the variables that differentiated dates in which sexual aggression occurred from dates involving the same respondents without aggression (Muehlenhard and Linton, 1987).

These studies provide some evidence that the habitual use of alcohol is associated with sexual victimization, but they do not explain the causal pathways. The evidence suggests that alcohol abuse is an aftereffect of earlier victimization, but the effect that alcohol might have on future victimization is unclear. Alcohol may directly increase the risk of victimization through cognitive and motor impairment that prevents women from recognizing, escaping, or resisting sexual aggression (Nurius and Norris, 1996). Studies of the cognitive effects of alcohol on victims parallel efforts to examine the social information processing of offenders. Rape victims who were drinking report that their judgment was impaired at the time of assault (Frintner and Rubinson, 1993).

It is possible, however, that the effect of alcohol is less direct. Drinking may increase the likelihood of victimization by placing women in settings in which their chances of encountering a potential offender are higher than the average. Several studies have suggested that bar settings increased women's vulnerability to violence independent of the increased vulnerability due to alcohol consumption. For example, exposure to obnoxious behavior, as well as sexual and physical violence, were predicted by the frequency of going to bars (Fillmore, 1985; Lasley, 1989). Alternatively, alcohol consumption by women may be misperceived and misinterpreted by the men they meet as a sexual availability cue. Although scientific evidence suggests that women become less physiologically aroused after drinking, men perceived them as more sexual, more likely to initiate sexual intercourse, and more aroused by erotica (Crowe and George, 1989; George et al., 1990, 1995; Corcoran and Thomas, 1991). In one study, 75 percent of college men admitted to getting a date drunk or high on drugs to try to have sex with her (Mosher and Anderson, 1986).

CONSEQUENCES

The consequences of violence against women are far broader than the impact on the women victims. Their families and friends may be affected. In the case of intimate partner violence, there is increasing evidence of the negative impact on children of exposure to violence in the family. Society suffers economically, both in the use of resources and in the loss of productivity due to fear and injury. Understanding the consequences of violence is necessary for planning and implementing interventions to deal with those consequences. This section examines research findings about the consequences violence against women has on the individual victim, those closest to her, and on society as a whole.

Consequences to Victims

Research in recent years has brought an increased understanding of the impact of trauma, in general, and of violence against women, in particular. Both rape and intimate partner violence are associated with a host of short- and long-term problems, including physical injury and illness, psychological symptoms, economic costs, and death. It should be noted that part of what is known about the consequences of violence against women comes from studies of women who were seeking help, so it may not be representative of all victims. It is possible that these women suffered more severe trauma than women who do not seek help, and so represent the worst cases. The opposite is also possible: that women who come forward have suffered less fear and damage to their self-esteem, and therefore the worst cases remain hidden. Women who agree to participate in research may come from different social, ethnic, and economic backgrounds than those who do not participate. Finally, researchers do not always have the understanding or the resources to reach subgroups of victims who may either be at high risk for violence or face special challenges in recovery.

Virtually absent from the research are studies addressed specifically to the experiences of older women, disabled women, immigrant and refugee women, migrant farm worker women, rural women, Asian American women, American Indian women, homeless women, lesbian and bisexual women, drug-addicted women, and institutionalized women (Eaton, 1995; Gilfus, 1995). Whether or not these groups differ in the overall level of violence they experience, the evidence suggests that the descriptive characteristics of the assaults are very similar (Torres, 1991; Wyatt, 1992). However, the same act can have very different meanings depending on many features that shape perceptions and behavior, including the age of the victim, her relationship with the perpetrator, culture, social class, sexual orientation, previous history of violence, perceived intent of the violence, and perceived causes and effects of the violence (Murphy and O'Leary, 1994). Victims from oppressed racial, ethnic, or cultural groups or who are lesbian or bisexual face additional challenges that may influence their strategies and resources for recovery (Brown and Root, 1990; Sue and Sue, 1990; Wyatt, 1992; Garnets and Kimmel, 1993; Schriver, 1995). Most studies of the consequences of violence look at impairments; only a few studies examine resilience and strengths as protectors against untoward outcomes or as alternative results to impairment (Gilfus, 1995).

Also missing in the literature is a developmentally oriented approach that follows the outcomes of exposure to violence into later stages of adult development. Little is known of the impact of trauma on social roles, life patterns, and timing of life transitions. A life-span perspective would look at differential effects on women's lives when violence involves multiple types and perpetrators, is ongoing, cumulative, and becomes a chronic feature of the environment. Many social and public health consequences of violence are unstudied, including labor force participation, economic well-being, fertility decisions, divorce rates, and health status (Gilfus, 1995).

Physical Consequences

Rape and Sexual Assault Surveys of adult females have found that women characterize the "typical" rape as entailing a high risk of physical injury and of death (Warr, 1985; Gordon and Riger, 1989). However, the data show that between one-half and two-thirds of rape victims sustain no physical injuries (Beebe, 1991; Koss et al., 1991; Kilpatrick et al., 1992); and only about 4 percent sustain serious physical injuries (Kilpatrick et al., 1992). Genital injuries are more likely in elderly victims (Muram et al., 1992). It appears that very few homicides are associated with rape: in 1993 only 106 of the 5,278 female homicide victims were also raped (Federal Bureau of Investigation, 1993). Even though serious physical injury is relatively rare, the fear of injury or death during rape is very real. Almost one-half of rape victims in a recent national study (Kilpatrick et al., 1992) feared serious injury or death during the attack. Rape can also result in transmission of a sexually transmitted disease (STD) to the victim, or in pregnancy. STD infection has been found in up to 43 percent of rape victims (Jenny et al., 1990), with most studies reporting STD infection rates between approximately 5 and 15 percent depending on diseases screened for and type of test used (Lacey, 1990; Murphy, 1990; Beebe, 1991). The rate of the human immunodeficiency virus (HIV) transmission due to rape is unknown (Koss et al., 1994), but it is of concern to a sizable proportion of rape victims (Baker et al., 1990). Pregnancy is estimated to result from approximately 5 percent of rapes (Beebe, 1991; Koss et al., 1991).

Rape has health effects that extend beyond the emergency period. Self-report and interview-administered symptom checklists routinely reveal that victims of rape or sexual assault experienced more symptoms of physical and psychological ill health than nonvictimized women (Waigant et al., 1990; Koss et al., 1991; Golding, 1994; Kimerling and Calhoun, 1994). Sexual assault victims, compared with nonvictimized women, were more likely to report both medically explained (30 percent versus 16 percent) and medically unexplained symptoms (11 percent versus 5 percent). Consequently, rape and sexual assault victims also seek more medical care than nonvictims. In longitudinal data, rape victims seeking care at a rape crisis center were initially similar to matched nonvictims in their self-reported physician visits, but at 4 months and 1 year after the rapes they were seeking care more frequently (Kimerling and Calhoun, 1994). These findings are consistent with studies using population data on medical use: women in primary care populations with a history of severe sexual and physical assault had nearly twice as many documented physician visits a year as nonvictimized women (6.9 versus 3.5; Koss et al., 1991). Utilization data across 5 years preceding and following victimization ruled out the possibility that the victims had been high users of services prior to their attacks.

A number of long-lasting symptoms and illnesses have been associated with sexual victimization including chronic pelvic pain; premenstrual syndrome; gastrointestinal disorders; and a variety of chronic pain disorders, including headache, back pain, and facial pain (for reviews see Koss and Heslet, 1992; Dunn and Gilchrist, 1993; Hendricks-Mathews, 1993). Persons with serious drug-related problems and high-risk sexual behaviors were also characterized by elevated prevalence of sexual victimization (Paone et al., 1992). These findings suggest that victimized women may become inappropriate users of medical services by somaticizing their distress; however, the number of sexual assault victims who qualify for the psychiatric diagnosis of somatization disorder is small. In a comparison of sexual assault victims with matched nonvictimized women on nine psychiatric diagnoses and a sample size of more than 3,000, too few cases of somatization disorder were identified to analyze statistically (Burnam et al., 1988).

Intimate Partner Violence   A woman is more likely to be injured if she is victimized by an intimate than by a stranger (Bachman and Saltzman, 1995). Victims of battering suffer from a host of physical injuries, from bruises, scratches, and cuts to burns, broken bones, concussions, miscarriages, stab wounds, and gunshot wounds to permanent damage to vision or hearing, joints, or internal organs to death. Bruises and lacerations to the head, face, neck, breasts, and abdomen are typical. Review of emergency room medical records in one urban hospital revealed that 50 percent of all injuries to women seen in the emergency room and 21 percent of the injuries that required emergency surgery could be attributed to battering. The review also found that 50 percent of the rapes of women over age 30 had been committed by the woman's intimate partner (Stark et al., 1981). Victims of partner violence were 13 times more likely to have injuries to the breast, chest, or abdomen than were accident victims (Stark et al., 1979), and three times as likely as nonbattered women to sustain injuries while pregnant (Stark and Flitcraft, 1988). Assaults directed at the abdomen can be associated with injuries both to the victim and the fetus (Helton et al., 1987a,b). In a representative national sample, 15 percent of pregnant women were assaulted by their partners at least once during the first half of pregnancy and 17 percent during the latter half (Gelles, 1988). A study of women attending prenatal clinics also found 17 percent of them suffered physical or sexual abuse during pregnancy (McFarlane et al., 1992). Several studies have found that white women experience more abuse during pregnancy than African American or Hispanic women (Berenson et al., 1991; McFarlane et al., 1992).

Women involved with a violent partner may be frequent users of medical services even if they do not identify the reason for their visit as the violence. They are likely to show evidence of injuries in various stages of healing, indicating the ongoing nature of the abusive behavior (Burge, 1989). Among women patients in a community-based family practice clinic who were living with a partner, recently separated, or divorced, 25 percent were assaulted by their partners during the previous year, and 15 percent sustained injuries from a partner (Hamberger et al., 1992). Some of this violence is lethal. Between 1976 and 1987, 38,468 people were killed by their intimate partners; 61 percent involved men who killed women. Among white couples, 75 percent of the victims were women (Browne and Williams, 1989, 1993).

Psychological Consequences

Victims of intimate partner violence and rape exhibit a variety of psychological symptoms that are similar to those of victims of other types of trauma, such as war and natural disaster. Following a trauma, many victims experience shock, denial, disbelief, fear, confusion, and withdrawal (Burgess and Holmstrom, 1974; Walker, 1979; Browne, 1987; Herman, 1992; Janoff-Bulman, 1992; van der Kolk, 1994). Assaulted women may become dependent and suggestible and have difficulty undertaking long-range planning or decision making (Bard and Sangrey, 1986). Although a single victimization may lead to permanent emotional scars, ongoing and repetitive violence is clearly highly deleterious to psychological adjustment (Follingstad et al., 1991). In one national study, the more a woman had been assaulted, the more psychological distress she experienced (Gelles and Harrop, 1989).[1]

A large empirical literature documents the psychological symptoms experienced in the aftermath of rape (for reviews see Frieze et al., 1987; Resick, 1987, 1990; McCann et al., 1988; Roth and Lebowitz, 1988; Hanson, 1990; Lurigio and Resick, 1990). Rape (with the exception of marital rape) is more likely than partner violence to be an isolated incident, which creates a somewhat different course of recovery. For many victims, postrape distress peaks approximately 3 weeks after the assault, continues at a high level for the next month, and by 2 or 3 months later recovery has begun (Davidson and Foa, 1991; Rothbaum et al., 1992). Many differences between rape victims and nonvictimized women disappear after 3 months with the exception of continued reports of fear, self-esteem problems, and sexual problems, which may persist for up to 18 months or longer (Resick, 1987). Approximately one-fourth of women continue to have problems for several years (Hanson, 1990).

Women who have sustained sexual or physical assault have been found to disproportionately suffer from depression, thoughts of suicide, and suicide attempts (Hilberman and

Munson, 1978; Hilberman, 1980; Kilpatrick et al., 1985; Stark and Flitcraft, 1988; McGrath et al., 1990; Dutton, 1992a,b; Herman, 1992). In one community sample, 19 percent of rape victims had attempted suicide in comparison with 2 percent of nonvictims (Kilpatrick et al., 1985). In other studies, 13 percent of rape victims suffered from a major depressive disorder sometime in their life, compared with only 5 percent of nonvictims (Burnam et al., 1988; Sorenson and Golding, 1990). Depression scores for victims of intimate partner violence on a widely used epidemiological measure (Radloff, 1977) were twice as high as the standard norms and well above the high-risk cutoff scores (Walker, 1984).

Other psychological symptoms reported by both victims of rape and partner violence include lowered self-esteem, guilt, shame, anxiety, alcohol and drug abuse, and posttraumatic stress disorder (PTSD) (Walker, 1979; Burnam et al., 1988; Winfield et al., 1990; Herman, 1992). Even when evaluated many years after they were sexually assaulted, survivors were more likely to receive several psychiatric diagnoses, including major depression, alcohol abuse and dependence, drug abuse and dependence, generalized anxiety, obsessive-compulsive disorder, and PTSD (Kilpatrick et al., 1985; Burnam et al., 1988; Winfield et al., 1990). Women who were both beaten and sexually attacked by their partners were at particular risk of the most severe psychological consequences (Shields and Hanneke, 1983; Pagelow, 1984; Browne, 1987).

There are few reliable predictors of positive readjustment among rape survivors (Hanson, 1990; Lurigio and Resick, 1990). In general, those assaulted at a younger age are more distressed than those who were raped in adulthood (Burnam et al., 1988). Some research has suggested that Asian and Mexican American women have more difficult recoveries than do other women (Williams and Holmes, 1981; Ruch and Leon, 1983; Ruch et al., 1991). Victims of these ethnic backgrounds, as well as Moslem victims, face cultures in which intense, irremediable shame is linked to rape. However, recent direct comparisons have revealed no ethnic differences in the psychological impact of rape as measured by self-report and interview-assessed prevalence of mental disorders among Hispanic, African American, and white women (Burnam et al., 1988; Wyatt, 1992).

The actual violence of an attack may be less important in predicting a woman's response than the perceived threat (Kilpatrick et al., 1987). The fear that one will be injured or killed is equally as common among women who are raped by husbands and dates as among women who are raped by total strangers (Kilpatrick et al., 1992). Likewise, acquaintance rapes are equally as devastating to the victim as stranger rapes, as measured by standard measures of psychopathology (Koss et al., 1988; Katz, 1991). However, women who know their offender are much less likely to report the rapes to police or to seek victim assistance services (Stewart et al., 1987; Golding et al., 1989). The impact of rape may be moderated by social support (Ruch and Chandler, 1983; Sales et al., 1984). Unsupportive behavior, by significant others in particular, predicts poorer social adjustment (Davis et al., 1991), and proceeding with prosecution appears to prolong recovery (Sales et al., 1984).

One way of systematizing some of the psychological responses evidenced by women victims of partner assault and rape is the diagnostic construct of posttraumatic stress disorder (PTSD) (Burge, 1989; Kemp et al., 1991; Dutton, 1992a). This construct has been used to understand a range of psychological responses to traumatic experiences, from natural disaster or military combat to rape and other forms of criminal attack (Figley, 1985; van der Kolk, 1987; Herman, 1992; Davidson and Foa, 1993). On the basis of clinical and empirical inquiries, a growing number of clinicians now suggest that PTSD may also be the most accurate diagnosis for many survivors of interpersonal and family violence (Herman, 1986, 1992; Bryer et al., 1987; van der Kolk, 1987; Burge, 1989; Gondolf, 1990; Koss, 1990; Davidson and Foa, 1991; Kemp et al., 1991; Koss and Harvey, 1991; Walker, 1991, 1992; Browne, 1992; Dutton, 1992a).

As early as 1974, Burgess and Holmstrom described what they termed "rape trauma syndrome" to describe the psychological aftermath of rape. Today, many assaulted women, like other victims of trauma receive diagnoses of PTSD. Among victims of intimate partner violence recruited from shelters and therapist referrals, 81 percent of those who had experienced physical attacks and 63 percent of those who had experienced verbal abuse were diagnosed with PTSD. Most rape victims (94 percent) who are evaluated at crisis centers and emergency rooms meet the criteria for PTSD within the first few weeks of the assault, and 46 percent still do so 3 months later (Rothbaum et al., 1992). Rape and physical assault are both more likely to lead to PTSD than other traumatic events affecting civilians, including robbery, the tragic death of close friends or family, and natural disaster (Norris, 1992).

Although the concept was initially constructed to explain reaction patterns in survivors of natural disasters and combatants in war, it is not surprising to find a high prevalence of PTSD among survivors of intimate violence. The most common trauma suggested for PTSD in the *Diagnostic and Statistical Manual of Mental Disorders* (American Psychiatric Association, 1994:427) is "a serious threat to one's life or physical integrity; [or] a serious threat or harm to one's children . . .," experiences known to characterize the lives of women in relationships with violent mates. Factors most often associated with the development of PTSD include perception of life threat, threat of physical violence, physical injury, extreme fear or terror, and a sense of helplessness at the time of the incident (March, 1990; Herman, 1992; Davidson and Foa, 1993). Moreover, some researchers suggest that PTSD is most likely to develop when traumatic events occur in an environment previously deemed safe (Foa et al., 1989), another dimension clearly applicable to violence occurring in one's home.

Many of the psychological aftereffects of violence against women can be understood as elements of a PTSD diagnosis (but see below). The PTSD construct has the advantage of providing a framework for recognizing the severe impact of events external to the individual (van der Kolk, 1987; Herman, 1992). However, for reactions to be seen as expectable responses to severe stressors, the trauma must be known. Unfortunately, in most mental health settings, routine screening for a history of family violence is almost never done; thus, serious or chronic psychological and physical conditions are treated without knowledge of the core trauma that may underlie current symptoms.

Finally, PTSD sufferers can become aware of the potential links between the symptoms that plague them and the exposure to an extreme external stressor. Clinical researchers consistently note how abused women internalize the derogatory attributions and justifications of the violence against them (Walker, 1979, 1984; Pagelow, 1984; Browne, 1987). An enhanced understanding of the range of responses manifested by all types of people who are faced with physical or sexual danger or attack expands the interpretation of symptoms beyond internal or gender explanations and empowers both survivors and providers to proceed with focused goals of safety, symptom mastery, reintegration, and healing (Herman, 1992).

Yet there are problems with the PTSD conceptualization. First, it doesn't account for many of the symptoms manifested by victims of violence. For example, thoughts of suicide and suicide attempts, substance abuse, and sexual problems are not among the PTSD criteria. Second, the diagnosis better captures the psychiatric consequences of a single victimization than the consequences of chronic abusive conditions (Herman, 1992). Third, the description of traumatic events as outside usual human experience is not accurate in describing women's experiences with intimate violence. Fourth, the diagnosis fails to acknowledge the cognitive effects of this kind of violence. People who have been untouched often maintain beliefs (or schema) about personal invulnerability, safety, trust, and intimacy, that are incompatible with the experience of violence (McCann and Perlman, 1990; Norris and Kaniasty, 1991).

In recent years, the notion of a battered woman syndrome has been used in a variety of legal proceedings, including criminal prosecutions of batterers, criminal prosecutions of women who have attacked their batterers, and divorce and child custody proceedings. The idea of the battered woman's syndrome developed as an attempt to explain the psychological effects of being in a battering relationship and has similarities with the PTSD conceptualization, but it is not a recognized psychiatric syndrome. Rather, it refers to the consequences of being battered as those consequences are represented in expert testimony in legal settings. The use of "battered woman syndrome" has been criticized for making those consequences of intimate partner violence for women a pathology and ignoring differences among battered women's responses to violence (e.g., Dutton, 1993, Schopp et al., 1994). Furthermore, because expert testimony about the experiences of battered women often encompasses more than just a discussion of psychological consequences, the term battered woman syndrome is misleading (Dutton, 1993).

Consequences to Family and Friends

Children in families in which the woman is battered are at risk of both physical (Walker, 1984; Straus and Gelles, 1990) and sexual abuse (Herman and Hirschman, 1981; Paveza, 1988). Even if children are not themselves abused, living in a family in which there is violence between their parents puts children at risk. These children have been found to exhibit high levels of aggressive and antisocial, as well as fearful and inhibited, behaviors (Jaffe et al., 1986a; Christopherpoulos et al., 1987). Other studies have shown that children who have experienced parental violence have more deficits in social competence (Jaffe et al., 1986b; Wolfe et al., 1986) and higher levels of depression, anxiety, and temperament problems than children in nonviolent homes (Jaffe et al., 1986b; Christopherpoulos et al., 1987; Holden and Ritchie, 1991). Jaffe et al. (1990) also found that children exposed to family violence see violence as an acceptable and useful means of resolving conflict.

Interpreting these findings should be done with caution. Not only is there debate about what constitutes exposure to violence (e.g., actually seeing the violent acts or seeing the results of the violence), but some of the studies have methodological weaknesses. For example, samples are often drawn from among children residing in shelters for battered women. These children are under a lot of stress—beyond that of witnessing violence—related to dislocation and family crisis that may influence their behaviors and feelings. The source of the information may influence the findings; mothers report more behavior problems in children than children self-report (Sternberg et al., 1993). However, these studies suggest that children exposed to parental violence are at potential risk of emotional and behavioral difficulties that may be long lasting.

Depression, developmental problems, acute and chronic physical and mental health problems, and aggressive or delinquent behavior are characteristic of children exposed to battering. An unknown number of the 3 million children exposed to battering each year (Jaffe et al., 1990) end up in foster care. Increased costs for schools, counseling, and juvenile justice programs have not been calculated. There are also unknown long-term costs associated with young boys who are learning how to be future batterers by modeling their fathers' behavior.

Longitudinal investigations that are both labor intensive and expensive are an important way to investigate how witnessing violence between one's parents during childhood is related to violence in one's own intimate relationships during adulthood. Widely cited assertions of intergenerational relationships in intimate partner violence are based on cross-sectional studies, and the findings are open to multiple explanations, including biases inherent in self-report data. There is evidence that longitudinal research following child victims may be needed to overcome possible problems with forgetting of childhood experiences (L. M. Williams, 1994).

Physical and sexual assaults may also affect other family members and friends, making them into secondary victims. Davis and colleagues (1995) found that rape, attempted rape, and aggravated assault of women all had negative psychological consequences on their friends, family members, and romantic partners, regardless of the victim's level of distress. Female friends and family members were more affected than male friends and family members, particularly in regard to increased fear of violent crime. Some rape victims also experience sexual dysfunction and difficulties with interpersonal relationships, both of which can have negative effects on their family relationships. Sexual dysfunction may be long lasting: Burgess and Holmstrom (1979) found that 30 percent of rape victims reported that their sexual functioning had not returned to normal as long as 6 years after the assaults.

Consequences to Society

Fear of Crime

Criminologists recognize that one social consequence of crime that affects many people beyond those who have been directly victimized is fear of crime (Hindelang et al., 1978; Skogan and Maxfield, 1981). The consequences of fear of crime are real, measurable, and potentially severe (Conklin, 1975; Skogan and Maxfield, 1981). Because women fear crime more than men (Warr, 1985; Gordon and Riger, 1989; Federal Bureau of Investigation, 1991), these consequences are disproportionately borne by women.

Women's fear of crime seems to be driven primarily by their fear of rape (Warr, 1985; Gordon and Riger, 1989; Klodawsky and Lundy, 1994; Softas-Nall et al., 1995). Women perceive rape as a very serious crime—at least as serious, if not more so, than murder (Warr, 1985; Softas-Nall et al., 1995).

The perceived risk of being raped is also high. Warr (1985) found young, urban women believed they were three times as likely to be raped as murdered and equally as likely to be raped as to suffer a less serious offense, such as theft of an auto. Similar ratings of seriousness and a high perceived risk of rape have been found in studies of women in Canada (Gomme, 1986), Great Britain (Smith, 1989), Germany (Kirchhoff and Kirchhoff, 1984), Holland (Van Dijk, 1978), and Greece (Softas-Nall et al., 1995). All these studies also found that women curtail their activities because of this fear: 42 percent of women in Warr's (1985) sample avoided going out alone (compared with only 8 percent of men), and 27 percent of women even refused to answer their door in response to fear.

Economic Effects

Existing data give some indication of the social consequences and attendant costs of violence. Straus (1986) estimated that intrafamilial homicide cost $1.7 billion annually; Meyer (1992) calculated the medical costs and lost work productivity of domestic violence at $5 to $10 billion per year; and the Bureau of National Affairs (1990) estimated the annual cost of domestic violence to employers for health care and lost productivity at $3 to $5 billion. Though alarming, the limited data available on women victims of violence and exclusion of sexual violence from these studies suggest that these figures may significantly underestimate the economic toll of violence.

It is estimated that between 12 percent and 35 percent of women visiting emergency rooms with injuries are there because of battering (Randall, 1990; Abbott et al., 1995). Outside of emergency departments, there is practically no information on a myriad of other health costs related to battering and sexual assault, such as treatment for depression and PTSD, drug and alcohol abuse, prenatal complications, suicide attempts, and other chronic physical and psychological conditions.

Estimates of the number of women who are homeless because of battering range from 27 percent (Knickman and Weitzman, 1989) to 41 percent (Bassuk and Rosenberg, 1988) to 63 percent of all homeless women (D'Ercole and Struening, 1990). In New York City, homeless shelters cost $125-130 per day per family; battered women's shelters with a variety of services cost more than $200 a day (Lucy Friedman, personal communication). But there is little information about other social service costs resulting from battering, such as the number of women and children on welfare because of abuse or the total costs of providing battered women with job training and placement, victim assistance services, and child care.

Battering and sexual assault puts an enormous burden on the criminal justice system; a study in the District of Columbia found that 22 percent of 911 calls were from victims of battering (Baker et al., 1989). Yet the full extent of costs to the courts—civil and family, as well as criminal—and law enforcement generally have not been calculated. These include costs associated with getting and enforcing orders of protection; divorce, child custody, and support proceedings; and prosecutions for assault, sexual assault, stalking, trespassing, harassment, and murder, all of which involve personnel costs for prosecutors, judges, defense lawyers, court staff, and police, among others. In addition, anecdotal evidence suggests that some battered women may be forced into performing criminal acts by their batterers (Browne, 1987).

Indirect Costs

Researchers are just beginning to look at the indirect costs of battering and sexual assault—costs that result not from using services but from reduced productivity and changes in quality of life. For example, a study by Victim Services in New York City found that 56 percent of working battered women had lost a job as a direct result of the violence, and 75 percent had been harassed while they were at work by their partners (Friedman and Couper, 1987). Resick et al. (1981) found women's work performance to suffer up to 8 months after rape. The costs of such reduced productivity or of constricted opportunity are unknown. How many women are prohibited from working by jealous partners or cannot concentrate at work because of battering or sexual assault? How many days are missed by women embarrassed to come to work with a black eye, afraid that the batterer will harass them at the office, or fearful of leaving their homes after being raped? Do partners or family members of rape victims lose time from work because of caring for injured victims or accompanying them to court?

Diminished quality of life is another unexplored indirect cost. What are the costs associated with the isolation, fear, and lack of freedom that plague the lives of battered women and their children? How many activities and opportunities do women forsake out of fear of sexual assault? What are the long-term costs to society of batterers'—and victims'—inability to parent their children? Information on the direct and indirect costs of violence against women would provide a useful guideline for evaluating the cost-effectiveness of intervention programs.

CONCLUSIONS AND RECOMMENDATIONS

Better understanding of the causes of violence against women will be useful in designing both prevention programs and interventions with offenders. Research has begun to identify childhood precursors to later violent aggressive behavior, and criminological research has studied the progression of criminal careers. Yet little research has considered the development of violence against women and whether pathways to violence against women are similar to the development of other violent behaviors. Nor is it known if physical and sexual violence against women develop in a similar manner and what the nature and extent of the relations among them are. Identifying precursors to violence against women may be important for early intervention and prevention efforts.

Most of the information on violence against women comes from either clinical samples or general population surveys. Clinical samples are most likely not representative of either victims or perpetrators; in general population surveys, the numbers of ethnic, racial, cultural, and other subgroups are too small for analysis. Differences among subgroups in the causes of violence against women could have important implications for prevention and intervention strategies. Subgroups about which information is lacking include racial and ethnic minorities, lesbians, migrant workers, immigrants, the homeless, the disabled, and the elderly.

Recommendation: Longitudinal research, with particular attention to developmental and life-span perspectives, should be undertaken to study the developmental trajectory of violence against women and whether and how it differs from the development of other violent behaviors. Particular attention should be paid to factors associated with the initial development of violent behavior, its maintenance, escalation, or diminution over time, and the influence of socioeconomic, cultural, and ethnic factors. Funding is encouraged for identification and analysis of existing data sets that include relevant information. In addition, research on the causes and consequences of violent behavior should include questions about violence against women.

Although some of the direct effects of physical and sexual violence (and psychological abuse) on individual women have been fairly well documented, understanding indirect effects to victims, the consequences to women in general, and consequences to the society as a whole is only beginning. Research suggests that women who have been victims of violence seek physicians' care not directly related to the violence nearly twice as often as other women. Some preliminary data indicate that intimate partner violence may play a role in women's need to receive and remain on welfare. As mandatory arrest laws continue to be passed, and as more jurisdictions encourage filing charges in cases of sexual assault, the criminal justice system faces increased costs. Some research on rape has found reduced job performance for up to 8 months after an assault. There is very little information on lost productivity and reduced performance, on the job and at home, of victims of violence.

Recommendation: Research is needed on the consequences of violence against women that includes intergenerational consequences and costs to society, including lost productivity and the use of the criminal justice, medical, and social service systems. Such research should address the effects of race and socioeconomic status on consequences of violence.

NOTE

1. In a national study of youths aged 10 to 16 years, more than one-third reported having been victims of sexual or physical assaults. This group revealed significantly more psychological distress including sadness and symptoms of posttraumatic stress disorder even after controlling for other variables that predict these outcomes (Boney-McCoy and Finkelhor, 1995). However, this study did not report outcomes separately for girls, who were far more likely to experience sexual assault, and boys, who experienced much more physical assaults by strangers. Nevertheless, the authors concluded that sexual assault in particular posed a very significant risk factor to the mental health of adolescents.

4

Prevention and Intervention

This chapter examines the types of responses society has made to violence against women. There are a number of ways to define and characterize prevention and intervention. This report uses one that best identifies the kinds of responses society can take and the research that can inform those responses. First, however, it notes several other classifications.

The public health perspective classifies "interventions" into primary, secondary, and tertiary prevention. The goal of primary prevention is to decrease the number of new cases of a disorder or illness. The goal of secondary prevention is to lower the prevalence of a disorder or illness in the population. The goal of tertiary prevention is to decrease the amount of disability associated with the disorder or illness. Although these three categories seem conceptually distinct, in practice there is disagreement over their use (Institute of Medicine, 1994). Another classification is Gordon's (1983, 1987) proposal for universal, selected, and indicated preventive measures. Universal preventive measures are desirable for everyone in a population; selected preventive measures are desirable for those in the population with an above average risk of acquiring a disorder; and indicated preventive measures are desirable for individuals who are identified as being at high risk for the development of a disorder. Because of frequent confusion over the meaning of the public health classifications, the Institute of Medicine (1994) recommended the use of a combination of it and Gordon's: preventive interventions, broken into three categories modeled after Gordon's; treatment intervention, which includes identification and standard treatments; and maintenance intervention, which aims at reducing relapse and recurrence and promoting rehabilitation.

This report adopts the Institute of Medicine's (1994) use of preventive interventions, but considers treatment and maintenance interventions together under the rubric of treatment interventions. Treatment interventions are separated into individual and community-level interventions: individual treatment interventions are those, such as counseling, that are targeted at the individual; community-level interventions represent more system-oriented interventions, such as criminal justice reforms, rape crisis centers, and battered women shelters. Following this classification, the chapter first discusses preventive interventions. Second, it considers treatment interventions, both the services available to women victims of violence and those, including criminal justice interventions, for offenders.

PREVENTIVE INTERVENTIONS

School-Based Preventive Programs

Preventive intervention efforts have largely consisted of school-based programs on conflict mediation, violence prevention in general, dating violence, sexual abuse, and spouse abuse. There are few data available on how widespread these programs are or to whom they are offered. Sexual assault and rape education programs seem to be increasingly common on college campuses; conflict resolution programs have been instituted in thousands of middle and high schools (Webster, 1993). The programs vary in length, in content, and in degree of theoretical underpinning. Evaluations are rare. The few evaluations that have been done of these programs generally test students' knowledge about and attitudes on relationship violence before and after the prevention program, as well as personal experience with dating violence (Jones, 1991; Jaffe et al., 1992; Kantor and Jasinski, 1995).

In Minnesota, the Minnesota Coalition for Battered Women developed a secondary school violence prevention program and trained secondary school teachers in the use of the curriculum. The approximately 200 teachers who were willing to participate in the evaluation were stratified by junior or senior high, and by rural, suburban, or urban location. Teachers were randomly selected from each of the six subgroups, and their students became the sample for the evaluation. Control groups from the same or nearby schools were also tested. Both groups were given preprogram and postprogram tests to assess their knowledge about battering, their attitudes, and their knowledge about the resources available for help in addressing relationship violence. Students who were given the 5-day prevention program improved their knowledge scores significantly more than the control group. However, attitudes among both experimental and control groups showed very little change. There was a posttest significant difference between girls' and boys' scores, with the girls' scoring more in the desired direction. The experimental groups also became more knowledgeable about general resources available for help with relationship violence, such as a hospital or mental health center, although they could not name specific local services (Jones, 1991).

Other studies have found attitudinal changes following school-based intervention programs. Students in four secondary schools in London, Ontario, were involved in a dating violence prevention program (Jaffe et al., 1992). The program involved a large group presentation followed by classroom discussion led by trained facilitators. Questionnaires were administered to 737 students—selected by means of stratified classroom-level sampling—both 1 week prior to the intervention and 1 week after; at two of the schools, a delayed posttest was also given 6 weeks after the program. Overall, the evaluation showed significant positive changes after intervention on knowledge, attitudes, and behavioral intention. A small group of males, however, showed change in an undesired direction.

Significant decreases in attitudes justifying the use of dating violence were found in a study of a prevention program in a Long Island, New York, high school (Avery-Leaf et al., 1995). The intervention consisted of five weekly sessions incorporated into a health class. The experimental group of 196 students were tested before and after the five-class program, and there was a control group of students whose health classes did not include the dating violence prevention program.

While all of these programs may change knowledge or attitudes about physical and sexual violence between intimates, no longitudinal studies exist to document whether they have any short- or long-term impact on the commission of dating violence, date rape, or intimate partner violence later in life. A review of evaluations of a broad array of prevention programs aimed at adolescents—including pregnancy prevention, drug abuse prevention, delinquency prevention— found that curricula that only provide information about risks and use scare tactics have little or no positive impact and may even result in more of the undesired behavior (Dryfoos, 1991; National Research Council, 1993). Intensive programs that include social-skill training and follow-up booster sessions may hold more promise, particularly if classroom efforts are part of a more comprehensive, community-wide strategy (Dryfoos, 1991; Webster, 1993).

Media Roles

Public education campaigns, such as those mounted against smoking and drunk driving, are a universal preventive intervention that have been part of other successful community prevention projects (Institute of Medicine, 1994). The Advertising Council, in conjunction with the Family Violence Prevention Fund, in June 1994 began a public education campaign against intimate partner violence. The campaign consists of television, radio, and print public service announcements "designed to increase public awareness of battering and to motivate individuals to take action to reduce and prevent abuse" (Family Violence Prevention Fund, 1995). The advertising campaign is being evaluated. A preadvertising survey that measured attitudes toward battering was conducted; there will be several postadvertising surveys that will look at advertisement recognition and changes in attitudes about battering, willingness to intervene in battering, and knowledge of community resources (Lieberman Research Inc., 1995).

Separate from public service announcements and other advertising, television programming has the potential to convey antiviolence messages. The recent National Television Violence Study (Mediascope, 1996) suggests that television could be used to send more prosocial messages about violence by showing the negative consequences of violent behavior and nonviolent alternatives to solving problems and by emphasizing antiviolent themes. There has been no research on the effects of such television programming.

Deterrence

To the extent that the threat of criminal justice sanctions deters people from engaging in violent behavior, they can be thought of as preventive interventions. The theory of deterrence is well established in the field of criminal justice (for reviews, see Zimring and Hawkins, 1971; Geerken and Gove, 1975; Gibbs, 1975; Cook, 1977; Blumstein et al., 1978; Tittle, 1980; Paternoster, 1987; Klepper and Nagin, 1989). The theory suggests that increasing the certainty of sanctions increases their deterrent effect (Reiss and Roth, 1993). From this perspective, mandatory arrest for intimate partner violence, increasing rates of prosecution for rape and intimate partner violence, and stricter enforcement of protection orders could be considered preventive interventions. (For a more complete discussion of these types of interventions, see the section on Criminal Justice Interventions, below.)

Other Issues in Rape Prevention

The literature on rape prevention includes strategies for rape avoidance and rape resistance, which are considered by some—particularly in the criminal justice field—to be prevention through reduction of opportunity. Rape avoidance entails strategies to be used by women to minimize their risk of sexual assault. These strategies include avoiding dangerous situations, not going out alone at night, keeping doors and windows closed and locked, and other precautions to be taken by women. Although these avoidance techniques may reduce a woman's risk of being sexually assaulted by a stranger, it is not clear they would reduce acquaintance attacks (Koss and Harvey, 1991). These strategies are also criticized as restricting women's activities and as potentially placing the blame on women who are sexually assaulted for not taking adequate precautions (Brodyaga et al., 1975, as cited in Koss and Harvey, 1991). The extent to which a woman chooses to use any particular avoidance strategy may depend on the importance she attaches to the perceived costs and benefits of the strategy (Furby et al., 1991). An emphasis on rape avoidance may actually increase the fear of rape (Koss and Harvey, 1991). Furthermore, avoidance strategies may do little to lower the overall rate of sexual assault; they may simply displace the assault from one potential victim to another.

Rape resistance strategies involve recommendations to women on what to do should they be attacked. Storaska (1975) popularized among law enforcement agencies the theory that women should remain passive in the face of an attack to avoid angering the attacker and increasing her risk of serious injury or death. The majority of the research on resistance strategies, however, suggests just the opposite. Women who actively resist attack are more likely to thwart rape completion without increasing their risk of serious injury (Javorek, 1979; Bart, 1981; Quinsey and Upfold, 1985; Levine-MacCombie and Koss, 1986; Siegel et al., 1989; Ullman and Knight, 1991, 1992). The success of resistance strategies also appears to be linked to situational factors, such as the proximity of others to the attack site, and offender traits (Koss and Harvey, 1991).

This report does not consider rape avoidance or rape resistance to be preventive interventions, the goal of which should be reduction in rates of perpetration. Some researchers also consider rape prevention to mean minimizing the psychological impact of sexual assault; this report considers that topic under interventions for victims, not as prevention.

INTERVENTIONS FOR VICTIMS

There is no universal system of services available to victims of battering or sexual assault; they vary from community to community. Interventions may occur in the criminal justice system, the health care system, the social service system, the mental health system, or some combination of systems. As noted above, the discussion of interventions is divided into those whose main focus is on the individual and those whose focus is institutional or community based; individual-level interventions seek to ameliorate the consequences of individual victimization; community-level interventions seek to change systems' responses to victims.

Individual-Level Interventions

Individual counseling and peer support groups are probably the services most used by battered women. A survey of 250 victims of battering in New York City who called 911 for help found that 43 percent of the callers wanted counseling services and 42 percent said they wanted someone to talk to about their feelings (Taylor, 1995). However, few data exist on how many battered women actually seek counseling services: of those seeking counseling services in the New York City study, Taylor (1995) found approximately two-thirds actually received them. Although specific therapy elements have been recommended for use with battered women (e.g., Walker, 1994), the panel found no evaluation studies of individual counseling or support groups for battered women.

Counseling services are also available for couples in which the woman has been battered or otherwise victimized, but there remains much debate in the field over the merits and advisability of couples counseling (Dobash and Dobash, 1992; Edleson and Tolman, 1992; Gondolf, 1993). Many practitioners and researchers argue that couples counseling is never appropriate when violence is present because it endangers women. Other counseling providers argue that couples counseling that is specifically designed to address the use of aggression may be beneficial for couples in discordant or mildly violent relationships (Pan et al., 1994; O'Leary et al., 1995). Because couples counseling is generally viewed as an intervention for the perpetrator, evaluations of it are addressed below in the section on interventions for batterers.

Mental health interventions with rape victims have received more study than those with battered women. Treatment approaches designed to address the postrape psychological consequences have been developed, and in some instances evaluations were undertaken to assess their effectiveness. However, in a review of the rape treatment outcome studies, Foa et al. (1993) concluded that few studies used an approach that would permit drawing conclusions about effectiveness. In most cases, there was no control group so it was not possible to determine whether improvements were a function of the passage of time or the intervention. The early studies that randomly assigned victims to different conditions produced mixed results. Veronen and Kilpatrick (1982) developed a brief, focused intervention implemented immediately post rape and designed to be prophylactic; they found that active treatment was no more therapeutic than assessment only. In contrast, a comparison of different six-session therapy approaches found that all three types of intervention produced improvement while victims on a naturally occurring waiting list did not improve (Resick et al., 1988).

Two more recently reported studies examined the effectiveness of specific treatments for victims suffering from posttraumatic stress disorder (PTSD). Foa and colleagues (1991) compared stress inoculation training—a combination of cognitive-behavioral and relaxation techniques to teach clients to control their fear, prolonged exposure—reliving the rape scene in the imagination in order to confront fear, and supportive counseling. They found that all treatments produced improvements at posttreatment, but at a 3-month follow-up, exposure appeared to be the most effective for PTSD symptoms. A cognitive processing approach designed to address maladaptive beliefs, as well as rape-related fears, reduced symptoms compared to a waiting-list control group (Resick and Schnicke, 1992). These studies support the conclusion that treatment for rape victims can be helpful and that specific types of treatment may be more effective for certain symptoms.

Community-Level Interventions

Crisis-Oriented Services: Shelters, Rape Crisis Centers, and Advocacy

A recent survey (Plichta, 1995) found 1,800 programs, of which approximately 1,200 were shelters, targeted at battered women in the United States. The programs offer a variety of services including hotlines, temporary shelter services, group and individual counseling, legal advocacy, social service referral and advocacy, services for children of abused women, transitional housing, child care, and job training. Public education and changing social norms with respect to battering are also an integral part of "the shelter movement." In addition to shelters, individual social workers, psychologists, and clinics that offer therapy and counseling services undoubtedly provide services to some victims of battering.

Little data exist on how many clients are served by the various programs or who those clients are. It does appear that the services are inadequate to meet the needs of all victims of battering who seek them. For example, in New York City in March 1995, about 300 women and children a week were denied emergency shelter due to lack of space (O'Sullivan et al., 1995).

There is some information on the women who do use shelter services. They tend to be from low socioeconomic groups, possibly because they have fewer resources available to them than women from higher socioeconomic groups. For example, in one study (O'Sullivan et al., 1995) 76 percent of the sample were on public assistance; another 1 percent had no income whatsoever. In another large sample of women using services in Texas (1,482 battered women in shelters and 650 battered women using nonresident shelter-based programs), Gondolf and Fisher (1988) found that a substantial portion lived in poverty. Over one-half of their sample had no personal income, and three-fourths of the women's husbands made less than $15,000 per year. The women who sought only nonresident services tended to be from higher socioeconomic groups than those who sought resident shelter services. In a sample from a shelter in a medium-sized Midwestern city, 81 percent of the women were receiving some type of government assistance, and 60 percent lived below the poverty line (Sullivan et al., 1994). It is often suggested that women with more economic resources may be able to pay for temporary shelter, for example at a hotel, and that they obtain other services through private means, such as individual counseling.

Shelter service seekers also have low educational attainment. In the Texas sample, about one-half of the women had not completed high school, and only about one-fifth had some post-high-school education (Gondolf and Fisher, 1988). Similarly, 45 percent of the New York sample had not finished high school, 31 percent had a high school diploma, and 23 percent had attended some college.

The racial characteristics of shelter users seem to depend on the location of the shelter. In Texas, 57 percent of the women were white, 15 percent were African American, and 29 percent were Hispanic. In New York City, 52 percent of shelter users were African American, 39 percent were Latina, and 9 percent were white or other (O'Sullivan et al., 1995). In the Midwestern sample, 45 percent of the participants were white, 43 percent African American, 8 percent Latina, and 1 percent Asian American (Sullivan et al., 1994). In preliminary data on shelters in the deep South, Donnelly and Cook (1995) found residents to be primarily white: only 2 of the 16 shelters they had surveyed (to date) targeted women of color. In recruiting a sample of abused women for a study in Newark, New Jersey, Joseph (1995) found more African American abused women in shelters for the homeless than in shelters for victims of battering. Since such characteristics as socioeconomic status, race, ethnicity, and educational level of all the women in a region who may need shelter services are not known, it cannot be determined if the shelter populations are representative of the battered women in an area.

Race and ethnic origin may be important factors in assessing the needs of women who use shelter services and in understanding barriers that may exist to obtaining services. For example, in comparison with white and African American women, Hispanic women in Texas shelters had been married the longest, had lower education, employment, and job status, and tended to report the longest duration of abuse, thereby experiencing more socioeconomic barriers to ending victimization (Gondolf and Fisher, 1988). There are few descriptions in the literature of programs that are successfully serving minority communities (Norton and Manson, 1997).

There has been little evaluation of the services offered to

battered women. Basic data on how many women and their children receive services, and the type of services received, are not available in any systematic form. Some state coalitions collect information from services within their state, but there is no uniform definition of what constitutes services. The Centers for Disease Control and Prevention of the U.S. Department of Health and Human Services is in the process of fielding an inventory of service availability and clientele served in order to develop some of this information.

Most studies of shelters and the outcome of shelter stays are descriptive. The panel's literature search found no experimentally controlled evaluations comparing outcomes for women using shelters with outcomes for women not using shelters. Some studies compare women's experiences preshelter stay to postshelter (Cannon and Sparks, 1989), compare groups of shelter residents based on services provided either during or after the shelter stay (Gondolf and Fisher, 1988; Cox and Stoltenberg, 1991; Sullivan et al., 1992, 1994), or compare shelter residents to women seeking other services (Berk et al., 1986). Recruiting samples of battered women to study can be quite difficult. Most of the studies have taken samples from women who seek help at a shelter or other service (for example, the courts). Using samples drawn from services makes it impossible to have a control group who has not sought services. Some researchers advertise for subjects through magazines, newspapers, or other media outlets. Although this method of recruiting may bring forth both women who have used shelter services and who have not, the sample is subject to self-selection bias. Of course, neither recruitment method produces a random sample.

In addition to the difficulty of a bias-free sample for study recruiting, researchers have not agreed on what outcome to measure. While all shelters probably have as an ultimate goal, a violence-free life for the women, many shelters' immediate goal is women's empowerment and support for them in whatever decisions they make. There currently is no clear way to measure empowerment. Many studies look at living

arrangements after a shelter stay as a proxy for violence, assuming no violence if the woman is no longer living with her
abuser. Other studies have asked shelter residents where
they planned to live following the shelter stay and used this
planned living arrangement as a proxy for the presence or
absence of violence. It is obviously easier and less expensive
to use planned living arrangement as an outcome measure
than to try to follow a large sample of women over time to
determine their actual living arrangements or the actual level
of violence in their relationships. And it is true that planning
to leave may be an important step in ending a violent relationship, whether or not the woman actually leaves after any
given shelter stay. However, Berk et al. (1986) argue that the
outcome measure should be amount of abuse at some extended follow-up period. They note that planned and actual
living arrangements differ and, furthermore, that leaving a
batterer does not ensure a violence-free life. For example,
Sullivan et al. (1994) found that more than one-fourth of the
women in their sample who had ended their relationships
with their abusers continued to be physically abused by them.
However, using amount of violence or abuse is also problematic as an outcome measure for programs aimed at victims,
because it depends on the behavior of offenders who were not
in the program. Some argue that it is unfair to judge a program on the basis of measures over which the program can
exert no control or influence. A relatively new tactic is to
measure stage of change in the women who are participating
in the program. An instrument for this measurement is under development (Brown, 1995).

Sullivan and colleagues (Sullivan and Davidson, 1991;
Sullivan et al., 1992, 1994) have carried out a longitudinal
study of women who have received shelter services, some of
whom were randomly assigned to receive follow-up advocacy
services. At 6 months postshelter stay, there were no significant differences in the level of violence being experienced
between those who had received advocacy services and those
who had not.[1] The 10 weeks of advocacy services did result

in certain positive outcomes for the women. Women who had received advocacy services were more likely to have made an effort to obtain other resources they needed. Overall, however, women in both groups experienced significantly less violence and fewer injuries than they had 6 months prior to entering the shelter, suggesting that their shelter stay was beneficial. They also reported significantly lower levels of depression, fear and anxiety, and emotional attachment to their batterers and increased feelings of personal control, an overall higher quality of life, and increased satisfaction with their social supports.

A study by Berk et al. (1986) also found that, for some women, shelters appeared to limit new incidents of violence in the 6 weeks following shelter stays. Specifically, women who were actively taking control of their lives, as evidenced by taking a number of help-seeking actions in addition to a shelter stay, were more likely not to be victimized again after a shelter stay. For other women—those who did not take other actions—the impact of the shelter stay was either neutral or even triggered retaliation by their abusers. The sample in this study consisted of 155 battered women in Santa Barbara County, California, drawn from women who went either to the local shelter or whose cases were referred to the county prosecutor's office. Statistical adjustments were made to compensate for the nonrandom assignment to experimental (shelter stay) and control (no shelter stay) groups.

Using where women planned to live after leaving the shelter (i.e., with the batterer or apart from him) as their outcome measure, Gondolf and Fisher (1988) investigated the prediction of living arrangement using service-related variables associated with economic independence, intervention decisions made, and number of shelter services used. The most influential predictors of planned living arrangements were having the batterer in counseling and the three economic independence variables. The batterers' being in counseling was the single strongest predictor of returning: 53 percent of the women whose batterers were in counseling planned to return to them, compared with only 19 percent of those whose batterers were not in treatment. Even the effect of having independent income was overshadowed by the effect of treatment for batterers: 16 percent of women with their own income planned to return to their batterers, compared with 38 percent of women with their own income and whose batterers were in counseling.

Using a pre- and post-quasi-experimental quantitative design, supplemented by in-depth interviews, Tutty (1995) assessed social support/isolation, stress/coping, and self-esteem of women who used shelter follow-up programs designed to assist women who had decided to live independently. Social workers from the programs visited women in their homes for 1-2 hours per week to provide counseling and advocacy services. These visits began immediately after the shelter stay and continued for 3 to 6 months. The women in the sample significantly improved their scores for appraisal support (the availability of someone to talk to about one's problems) as measured by the Interpersonal Support Evaluation List after 3 months in the follow-up program. There was also some evidence of an increase in self-esteem by the end of the program. Although the sample size was quite small, this study supports the positive impact of post-shelter services found by Sullivan et al. (1992, 1994).

Rape crisis centers have been providing services for victims for more than 20 years (Koss and Harvey, 1991). This specialized response evolved when rape victims could not expect that family, friends, or medical and legal systems would either understand the nature of their trauma or respond supportively. The grass roots rape movement took on the tasks of ensuring that victims had access to informed and sympathetic advocate-counselors to assist with the emotional consequences of rape and to deal with the appropriate systems. These centers also considered community education, system reform, and empowerment of women and victims to be central to their mission. As in the shelter movement, changing the larger social climate has been as important an activity as providing direct services to victims.

Research on rape crisis services is descriptive in nature, cataloguing the kinds of services offered (O'Sullivan, 1976; Gornick et al., 1983; Burt et al., 1984) or other characteristics of the programs (Harvey, 1985). Most such services consist of 24-hour crisis lines offering information and support, advocacy in the form of information about the medical and legal systems, accompaniment to medical and legal appointments or court appearances, and supportive postrape counseling. The counseling has often been offered as a group treatment. In many cases, the services have been delivered by trained volunteers, but increasingly mental health professionals supervise or carry out the counseling.

Although the provision of these services for rape victims has come to be standard fare in many communities, there has been no systematic assessment of their effectiveness in helping reduce victims' distress. And these programs may not lend themselves to conventional methods of evaluation, with individual victims using pre- and postintervention measures of distress or assignment to various treatment conditions. Given that virtually all rape victims experience initial distress and that the purpose of intervention is to alleviate that distress with a supportive response, it is not reasonable to impose such an expectation. However, the characteristics of programs perceived as highly effective by their communities and by experts in the sexual assault field have been described (Harvey, 1985). The elements include maintaining a commitment to both victim services and social change, having a cohesive philosophy regarding program values and action, and developing the capacity to change in response to self-evaluation or shifts in the community or societal climate.

Health and Criminal Justice Services

Interventions in the health sector usually involve the treatment of injuries incurred in a physical or sexual assault.

For intimate partner violence, emphasis has been on identification of battered women and appropriate referral (Council on Scientific Affairs, 1992). In addition, the American Medical Association (1992) has issued guidelines for physicians on identifying and treating victims of intimate partner violence (McAfee, 1995). In spite of increased attention by the medical profession to the issue of intimate partner violence in the past several years, it appears that violence is often overlooked or not documented as a cause of injury (e.g., Abbott et al., 1995). However, as noted in Chapter 2, documentation of abuse in medical records is not without potential costs to the victim, such as denial of health insurance coverage.

Besides treating the injuries of a sexual assault victim, a hospital emergency room is often critical to gathering forensic evidence to be used if legal charges are brought against an assailant. Sexual assault nurse examiner (SANE) programs have been established in some cities to provide comprehensive care to sexual assault victims (Ledray and Arndt, 1994). Although there may be variation, all forensic nursing examinations of sexual assault victims include five essential components: treatment and documentation of injuries; treatment and evaluation of sexually transmitted diseases; evaluation of pregnancy risk and prevention; crisis intervention and arrangements for follow-up; and collection of medical and legal evidence while maintaining the proper chain of evidence (Hazlewood and Burgess, 1995).

Most of the criminal justice system responses relate to sanctions for perpetrators of violence and so are discussed below. However, aspects of the criminal justice system can be thought of as interventions for victims. Victims of sexual assault and intimate partner violence often face barriers that keep them from making use of the criminal justice system. Battered women may be reluctant to involve the criminal justice system out of fear of retaliation and fear of the criminal justice system itself (e.g., Fischer and Rose, 1995). Victims of sexual assault may be reluctant to report their victimization out of fear of the stigma attached to sexual assault, fear of retaliation, and fear of the ordeal of court (e.g., Kilpatrick et al., 1992). Although there has not been much research, it appears that changes in the criminal justice system could improve women's experiences. Efforts to make the criminal justice system more responsive to victims' concerns are being tried in varous communities. Such efforts include reforming laws; training police, prosecutorial, and court personnel; creating special units to investigate sex crimes; and providing victim advocates to assist women through the criminal justice process. These efforts have not been widely studied.

Increasing access to the criminal justice system may benefit women in a number of ways—increasing women's safety, improving women's sense of self-efficacy, and making a statement about the community's intolerance of violence against women. The degree to which arrest or protective orders do or do not improve battered women's safety has yet to be resolved. (The research on arrest is discussed in more detail in the section on interventions with offenders.) Women are more likely to call the police and police are more likely to make an arrest for the first battering incident or if a battering incident results in injury (Bachman and Coker, 1995). Whether arrest of perpetrators makes battered women safer is still not known, but recent analysis indicates arrest does not increase their danger more than any other police intervention (Garner et al., 1995). Willingness of the police to arrest batterers may improve women's satisfaction with police response and increase their willingness to call on the police in the future (Jaffe et al., 1993).

Protective orders, both temporary and permanent, also appear to serve specific functions for women in addition to protecting them from their batterer. Based on in-depth interviews with women who had applied for protective orders, Fischer and Rose (1995) found that women felt protective orders told their batterers that society did not approve of their behavior. Getting a protective order also served as documentation of the abuse—making it a matter of public record should anything happen to the woman and serving as proof to police that she was serious about ending her abuse. Finally, taking the step of getting a protective order enhanced women's sense of self-efficacy and control. Although Fischer and Rose interviewed only 83 women in one midwestern city, their findings are suggestive of the ways in which criminal justice system interventions affect victims of violence.

Many of the reforms in rape laws were promoted as efforts to make it easier to prosecute and convict offenders (see discussion under interventions with offenders). Changes in rape shield laws, however, were predicted to make it easier for women to report rapes and less onerous for them to testify in court. (Rape shield laws determine how much of a victim's sexual history can be used as evidence in court.) The few studies that have looked at the impact of rape law reform have found no clear-cut evidence that rape shield laws had the intended effect (Horney and Spohn, 1991). There is evidence that the rate of reporting rape has increased nationally since the early 1970s, when rape laws began to be reformed (Bourque, 1989), but because of the variety of state laws, it is impossible to attribute that increase to legal reform. Furthermore, there are no good data on how often a complainant's sexual history had actually been used in cases prior to the enactment of rape shield laws (Horney and Spohn, 1991). Overall, a great deal of judicial discretion remains in deciding how much evidence about a victim's sexual history is allowed in court.

Other Services and Service Seeking

In order to better understand what services are important to battered women, Gondolf and Fisher (1988) studied a sample of 1,482 battered women in shelters and 650 battered women using nonresident shelter-based programs in Texas. They looked at seven categories of services offered to shelter residents: referral, transportation, medical care, child services, counseling, legal services, and employment services.

Gondolf and Fisher concluded that shelters play a pivotal role in facilitating help seeking. These women used the shelter for much more than just refuge. An average of 3.3 services were used: 45 percent of the Texas women used only one or two services, 37 percent used three or four services, and 20 percent used five, six, or seven services. The most used services were counseling (85 percent), transportation (73 percent), and referral (67 percent). On average, the women anticipated using two services after leaving the shelter; nearly one-third said they would use three or more services. The services they anticipated using the most were the crisis hotline (70 percent), counseling (61 percent), and referral services (52 percent).

Taylor (1995) surveyed 250 victims of battering in New York City who had called 911 for help. The most common services sought were help with seeking an order of protection (58.5 percent), counseling (43.1 percent), and discussion of troubling feelings (42 percent). Nearly 80 percent of those who wanted help with protection orders or other legal assistance received that help. Table 4.1 details the services sought and received by these battered women.

Various studies of rape victims reveal an important finding: a majority do not seek crisis or advocacy services or treatment in spite of service availability. Koss (1988) found that only 4 percent of college student victims had contacted rape crisis centers. In a study conducted by Kimerling and Calhoun (1994), victims were assessed prospectively over 1 year following their rapes. Although victims continued to experience more psychological symptoms than a comparison group of nonvictims, only one-fifth sought mental health treatment even though they had access to rape crisis services. This lack of use of service contrasts with an increased use of medical services during the period.

Treatment outcome studies report that among the victims serving as subjects, many had waited years to seek treatment. For example, in both the Koss (1988) and Kimerling and Calhoun (1994) studies, in spite of the fact that all of the

TABLE 4.1 Services Sought and Received by Victims of Battering in New York City Who Called 911

Service	Percentage Who Sought Service	Percentage Who Received Service[a]
Help with order of protection	58.5	79.3
Counseling	43.1	65.0
Discussion of troubling feelings	42.0	68.4
Help with other practical problems	36.5	55.6
Help with emotional and practical problems for both victim and perpetrator	26.9	36.4
Help with housing	25.0	30.8
Legal assistance	24.0	80.0

[a]Of those who sought the service.

SOURCE: Taylor (1995:Table D.2). Reprinted by permission of Victim Services.

victims met diagnostic criteria for PTSD, the average length of time since the assault was about 6 years.

The components and characteristics of a service response have been identified (Koss and Harvey, 1991) and are often available in many communities. Yet these services for rape victims are often not used, even though at least some of these victims continue to suffer from rape-related effects and the available treatment could be helpful. It would be important to understand the barriers and facilitators to seeking the current array of crisis intervention, advocacy, and treatment services, and determine whether there are other types of services that victims want. Devising strategies to provide early assistance to victims who have significant mental health consequences might prevent or reduce needless additional suffering. It may be that the most effective approaches to reaching and serving victims have yet to be identified or fully developed.

Similarly, the majority of battered women may not seek services. In New York City, it is estimated that less than 2 percent of all battered women go through the shelter system, which is the entry point for many services (Friedman, 1995). There is some evidence to suggest that women who seek shelter services experience more frequent victimization than nonservice seekers. In studies by Giles-Sims (1983) and Okun (1986), women in shelters reported an average of between 65 and 68 assaults per year. The National Family Violence Survey of 1985 found an average of 6 assaults per year for all victimized women in the sample, and 15.3 assaults per year for women who had sought shelter services (Straus, 1990a). Women in shelters may have quantitatively different experiences from those of nonservice seekers associated with the difference in frequency of assaults. Yet since most of what is known about battered women and battering comes from samples of women drawn from shelter populations, lack of information about women who do not seek services represents a major gap in knowledge about violence against women. For victims of both rape and battering, it is not known to what extent they do not know about services, are unwilling or uable to use them, or choose not to use them.

CRIMINAL JUSTICE INTERVENTIONS
WITH OFFENDERS

Throughout U.S. history, women's advocates have sought laws and law enforcement to prevent violence against women. The modern women's movement succeeded in bringing federal attention to the problem in the 1970s.[2] In 1984 the U.S. Attorney General's Task Force on Family Violence published recommendations for justice system action and for needed research on family violence, including battering against women. More recently, the Violence Against Women Act of the Violent Crime Control and Law Enforcement Act of 1994 promotes a number of efforts in the criminal justice arena, such as arrest of batterers and those who violate protective orders; coordination of police, prosecutor, and judicial responsibilities for battering cases; and coordination of computer tracking systems for communication among police, prosecutors, and courts.

The women's movement in the 1970s called not only for the creation of services for women who had suffered violent victimization, but also for the criminal justice system to treat rape and battering as it did other crimes. This call entailed pressure for changes in laws, particularly with respect to rape, and better enforcement of the laws pertaining to all forms of violence against women. Interest in treatment for sex offenders and batterers also grew during the 1970s and 1980s.

A growing body of research has examined the impact of criminal justice interventions. There is mixed evidence about the ability of various criminal justice interventions to protect individual women or change individual men's behavior. The impact on the rate of battering or sexual assault at the community level remains unknown. In discussing criminal justice responses, it must be remembered that there really is not a single criminal justice system in the United States; rather there are at least 51 models, determined by state and federal laws, and numerous other practices associated with local jurisdictions. In addition, one cannot discuss criminal justice interventions in terms of individual- and community-level interventions as did the previous section. Many of the rehabilitation and counseling efforts that would be individual-level interventions are tied to the criminal justice system— community-level interventions—for offenders. This section, therefore, first summarizes the research on interventions for batterers and sexual offenders and then summarizes the research on rehabilitation (treatment) efforts.

Batterers

Arrest

Whether or not police should arrest perpetrators on the scene of batterings tends to dominate the discussions of appropriate police interventions. Warrantless arrest has been the subject of extensive research to evaluate its effectiveness in preventing battering. The Minneapolis Domestic Violence Experiment pioneered the use of randomized designs to compare the consequences of arrest to alternative police actions (Sherman and Berk, 1984). In the Minneapolis experiment, police officers' discretion was replaced with randomized treatments of arrest, separation, or offering advice before leaving the victim and offender together. Arrest was found to result in a reduced chance of new violence within the next 6 months. These findings encouraged many jurisdictions across the country to institute either mandatory or presumptive warrantless arrest for battering cases.[3]

Attempts to replicate the Minneapolis findings have resulted in less clear-cut outcomes. Known collectively as SARP (the Spouse Assault Replication Program of the National Institute of Justice), experiments testing arrest and alternative police interventions were performed in Omaha, Nebraska (Dunford et al., 1990), Charlotte, North Carolina (Hirschel et al., 1992), Milwaukee, Wisconsin (Sherman et al., 1992), Dade County, Florida (Pate and Hamilton, 1992), and Colorado Springs, Colorado (Berk et al., 1992). Because the experimental designs differed among the sites, comparing results proved difficult and confusing. Recently, Garner et al. (1995) reanalyzed the data for comparative purposes and concluded that arrest was no better or worse than other police actions much of the time. When arrest did make a difference, it reduced the chance of new violence relative to alternative police treatments. Contrary to some interpretations, Garner et al. (1995) found no reliable evidence that arrest increases the likelihood of repeat violence; rather, it may be less effective in decreasing violence than other practices. However, if arrest is an option, one must wonder if the failure to arrest is perceived by a batterer as implicit permission to continue his violent behavior (Buzawa and Buzawa, 1990).

The experience with the arrest studies indicates how difficult it can be to convert even well-designed studies into policy recommendations. The initial Minneapolis findings were widely circulated and led to arrest policies in many jurisdictions, even after the replication studies were less supportive of arrest (Sherman, 1992). Making policy on the basis of one unreplicated study can be risky, but research is not the only impetus for policy. It may be that the Minneapolis results simply reinforced other social pressures at the time, such as successful lawsuits against police departments that had failed to respond to battering incidents.

As in evaluations of services for victims, controversies arise over what outcomes should be measured and how to measure them. One may wish to measure subsequent violence, but the use of official records may not give an accurate portrayal of new incidents of violence. Victims may not report repeat violence to police for a number of reasons, including dissatisfaction with the police handling of the case. Estimates from National Crime Victimization Survey data indicate that only 56 percent of battering incidents are reported to police (Bachman and Coker, 1995). Other research has estimated that as few as 7 percent to 14 percent of battering incidents are reported (Kantor and Straus, 1990). When victims are pleased with police response, they may be more likely to report repeat violence (Davis and Taylor, 1995). In either event, what is being measured is not repeat violence, but willingness to call the police. Reliance on interviews with victims may catch repeat incidents of violence that were not reported to police, but victims are often difficult to locate or may not want to be interviewed. For example, of the 330 cases in the Omaha experiment, 67 (20.3 percent) of the women did not complete initial interviews and an additional 21 women (6.4 percent) could not be located for 6-month follow-up interviews (Dunford et al., 1990). Another issue in outcome measurement is how long the follow-up period should be.

Apart from the question of specific prevention, it remains to be demonstrated that arrest is a general deterrent to battering. Williams and Hawkins (1989) analyzed perceptual data from males interviewed as part of the second National Family Violence Survey (Straus and Gelles, 1986) to test the relative effects of formal and informal controls on potential aggression. They found that the greatest deterrent effect was associated with informal controls implied by moral disapproval of assault and by social attachments. A lesser, but significant, general deterrent operated through the perceived risk of arrest. Assuming that the perceived risk is enhanced by knowledge of actual arrests when police respond to incidents of battering, one can expect a proarrest policy to inform and then deter men who would be inclined to batter. There may be differential deterrence effects of arrest among various groups of men. For example, the extremely high arrest and incarceration rate (for all crimes) among urban African American young men may make arrest less of a deterrent for them. Yet African American women are more likely than white women to call the police, and African American men are more likely than white men to be arrested (Bachman and Coker, 1995).

Prosecution

In jurisdictions that have not paid special attention to or were apparently not concerned about domestic violence, prosecution rates of battering cases typically have been low (Ford, 1983; Dutton, 1988). In jurisdictions that are supportive of criminal justice interventions for domestic violence, prosecution rates have been higher (Ford, 1993).

Whether a case begins through arrest or a victim-initiated complaint, it is the prosecutor's office that acts as the gatekeeper in bringing a case to the courts. There is great variety across the country in policies pertaining to prosecution of battering cases. Some jurisdictions encourage victim-initiated complaints, while others discourage or outright refuse to prosecute such cases. There is some evidence to suggest that allowing victim-initiated complaints serves a protective function for the victim. Ford (1993) found a decrease in violence of at least 47 percent for any victim-initiated complaint policy, according to victim interview reports of incidents before and after prosecution.

A major issue in prosecution is whether or not a victim should be allowed to drop the charges. In general, it has been assumed that prosecution can only protect victims under policies meant to keep victims in the criminal justice system while state power is used to control offenders (U.S. Attorney General's Task Force on Family Violence, 1984; Goolkasian, 1986; Lerman, 1986). Foremost among recommended policies is a "no-drop" policy, promoted as making it impossible for a defendant to pressure a victim to drop charges, thereby possibly protecting the victim from coercive violence (Lerman, 1981). Furthermore, a no-drop policy signifies that the prosecution is committed to acting against battering, which may serve as a general deterrent. Others argue that a no-drop policy disempowers victims who may be able to use the possibility of dropping charges to negotiate self-protective arrangements (Elliott et al., 1985; Ford, 1991). Findings from the Indianapolis Domestic Violence Prosecution Experiment revealed that a victim who was permitted to drop charges and whose defendant had been arrested on a warrant had the lowest chance of suffering new violence within 6 months of the case's being settled (Ford, 1993). There is an important difference between a policy of allowing charges to be dropped and the actual dropping of charges. Ford (1993) also found that women who were permitted to drop charges and did so were no better off than those whose cases were prosecuted under a no-drop policy.

Protective Orders

Protective orders include any of a number of court orders demanding that a potentially dangerous suspect stay away from an identified individual. Typical orders include restraining orders issued in the course of a civil matter, orders of protection issued at the request of a victim who feels endangered, and no-contact orders issued by a criminal court during its proceedings or as a condition of probation. The terms of a protective order can vary from no violent contact to no contact whatsoever with the petitioner, her friends, coworkers, etc. Orders may specify terms of child visitation or use of property. Most states today have criminalized the violation of protection orders and give police officers the authority to make warrantless arrests for their violation.

The Violence Against Women Act of 1994 created a new crime of crossing a state line to violate a protective order. The law also gives full faith and credit to protective orders, so that an order issued in one state must be enforced in another state. Whether or not this federal law improves the enforcement of protection orders will depend in large part on how local police coordinate with federal authorities in enforcement.

A few studies have addressed the effectiveness of protective orders in preventing violence. All are limited in their findings by problems in implementing and enforcing their terms. In multiple sites around the United States, Grau et al. (1984) found that, although victims felt protective orders to be effective, there was no difference in rates of victimization between those with and without orders. Indeed, the study revealed evidence that protective orders may aggravate violence when they are not enforced by the police. Buzawa and Buzawa (1990) report that samples of police in Massachusetts rarely arrested people even when they had probable cause to act against violations of protective orders. Harrell et al. (1993) found that protective orders in Denver and Boulder were effective for at least a year in preventing violence against the petitioners in comparison with victims without orders. In other respects, however, the orders were largely ineffective: 75 percent of offenders contacted the victims and 21 percent stalked them. As in other studies, arrest for violations was rare, and, thus, compromised the potential of a protective order for preventing violence.

Courts and Judicial Processing

Judges and judicial processing are the least studied aspects of criminal justice, yet judges' discretion and court procedures can have profound effects on the actions of other parts of the criminal justice system and on victim safety. For example, Ferraro (1989) found that judges in Phoenix were critical of police who made arrests under the department's presumptive arrest policy, and, therefore, police were reluctant to make arrests.

Judges' decisions can directly affect battering cases: judges can determine pretrial release conditions, such as whether or not a defendant should be released, how long he should be held prior to release, the nature and amount of bond, and whether a protective order should be issued. In victim-initiated cases, judges decide whether to issue a warrant for the man's arrest or a summons for his appearance. During the course of a trial, judges make decisions about continuances and the types of evidence that will be allowed. If a defendant is found guilty, judges often exercise considerable discretion in sentencing. Little research exists on the effects of these various judicial decisions. In response to low rates of prosecution for batterers, some jurisdictions have created special courts to deal with cases involving intimate partner violence. Although no evaluations have been completed on the effects of such courts, the Dade County (Florida) Domestic Violence Court is currently being evaluated using an experimental design to see if legal sanctions are more likely and more severe under this system and if victims and their children are safer (Fagan, 1996).

Court-mandated counseling for batterers is a popular option from the perspective of both victims and criminal justice practitioners. It satisfies victims' interests that batterers receive help and seems to give judges a feeling of constructive action to rehabilitate offenders. Hamberger and Hastings (1993) describe two primary types of court mandates. The first is pretrial diversion, whereby the batterer can have his arrest record cleared or the charge reduced on successful completion of treatment. The second is a direct court order to participate in treatment as part of a sentence imposed after conviction. Little research has been done on the effect of court mandates on treatment completion or on whether sanctions are imposed for noncompliance.

One study of court-mandated treatment found that men who completed the program were significantly more likely to have been in treatment by court order (Hamberger and Hastings, 1989). About two-thirds of the court-mandated treatment group completed treatment, compared with about two-fifths of men whose treatment was not court ordered. Saunders and Parker (1989) found that other factors may have also been at work. In their study, younger, less well-educated men were more likely to complete treatment if it was court ordered; men over 25 with college educations were more likely to complete treatment if it was voluntary. Saunders and Parker (1989) also looked at the type of court mandate. Although significant differences in rates of attrition from treatment were not found, there was a trend for those men with deferred prosecution to have greater completion rates.

Much remains unknown about the impact of court-mandated treatment. Of particular concern is the effect of court-mandated treatment on reducing violent behavior. A few studies have found lower recidivism (as measured by repeat arrests) among men whose treatment was court mandated in comparison with men who received other court sanctions (Steinman, 1990; Palmer et al., 1992; Syers and Edleson, 1992). However, Harrell (1991) found higher recidivism among men in court-mandated treatment than among those in a nontreatment group.

Coordinated Community Responses

As changes came about in various components of the criminal justice system, both battered women's advocates and their colleagues in the various parts of the justice system recognized a need for more coordinated efforts (Hart, 1995). Multiple models of coordinated community approaches have been developed, including community intervention projects, coordinating councils, community partnering, technical assistance projects, and community organizing. Community intervention projects have been the most evaluated of the various models. These projects involve a grassroots organization that sets up procedures with the local criminal justice agencies to establish and monitor policies related to battering, to be informed of batterers' arrests so that advocates can be provided to the battered woman to help her navigate the legal system and locate services for herself and her children, and to provide information on batterers' treatment options to the arrested man; see Brygger and Edleson (1987) for a full description of a coordinated intervention project.

Although initial evaluations seem to indicate that coordinated community efforts may decrease repeat violence, research is sparse. Gamache et al. (1988) retrospectively studied three communities in which community intervention projects had been established. Using archival police and court records, they found that the projects had a significant impact on increasing the levels of arrests for battering, convictions, and court mandates to treatment. In a comparison of cases of battering that occurred prior to the establishment of a coordinated community effort to those after it was established, Steinman (1990) found that arrests prior to the coordinated effort increased repeat violence, while police action, particularly arrest, in coordination with other criminal justice efforts deterred further violence. Syers and Edleson (1992) collected data on all woman abuse cases during a 13-month period in two police precincts in Minneapolis. Besides looking at official police and legal advocate records, they interviewed as many female victims as could be reached by telephone contact immediately following the police visit and 6 and 12 months later. At 12 months, they found a trend for the least repeat violence among men who were arrested and ordered to treatment, followed by the men who were arrested and not ordered to treatment, with the highest repeat violence among men who were not arrested.

Coordinated community responses that involve activities other than domestic violence programs and the criminal justice system have not been evaluated. Many practitioners recognize the need for interactions and coordination among various systems that might intervene with victims and offenders. The Violence Against Women Act of 1994 includes demonstration grants for coordinating domestic violence programs with the criminal justice system, the social service system, the health care and mental health systems, the education community, the religious community, the business community, and other pertinent community groups and activities.

Sex Offenders

Rape Statute Reform

While much of the effort in criminal justice surrounding batterers concerned better enforcement of existing laws, for rape much of the effort was directed at reforming the rape laws. These reforms were expected to make it easier to obtain convictions of sex offenders as well as to improve the victims' experience in court so that women would be more willing to report sexual assaults.

Before the mid-1970s, most states' rape laws required prompt reporting of the crime; corroboration by other witnesses; physical resistance by the victim; and cautionary instructions to the jury about the difficulty of determining the truth of a victim's testimony. Most of these state statutes also narrowly defined rape as sexual intercourse with a woman not one's wife by force or against her will (Bienen, 1980). Beginning in the mid-1970s and continuing throughout the 1980s, most states changed their rape laws in a number of ways, including: definition of acts included; gradation of offenses; focus on behavior of offender rather than consent of victim; inclusion of rape shield provisions; elimination of witness corroboration; elimination of prompt reporting; elimination of cautionary instructions; and elimination of marital exclusion.

Most states moved to a gender-neutral definition of rape that includes vaginal, anal, and oral penetration by body parts or other objects. For example, the federal code (18 U.S.C. § 2245) defines sexual act as:

> (A) contact between the penis and the vulva or the penis and anus, and for purposes of this subparagraph contact involving the penis occurs upon penetration, however slight; (B) contact between the mouth and the penis, the mouth and the vulva, or the mouth and the anus; or (C) the penetration, however slight, of the anal or genital opening of another by a hand or finger or by any object, with an intent to abuse, humiliate, harass, degrade, or arouse or gratify the sexual desire of any person.

Many states and the federal code have also dropped the term "rape" and substituted a series of graded offenses such as "aggravated sexual abuse (or assault)," "sexual abuse," and "abusive sexual contact" that more closely parallel other criminal offenses. The graded offenses are differentiated by aggravating circumstances, such as use of a weapon, and have different levels of penalties attached. The intent of replacing the single offense of rape with a series of graded offenses was to make it easier to obtain convictions. It was predicted that the availability of lesser appropriate offenses would mean more convictions through plea bargaining and through providing juries options of lesser charges. However, conviction rates do not seem to have improved subsequent to these definitional changes (Horney and Spohn, 1991).

Another major shift in rape law reform has been the move from focusing on the consent of the victim to focusing on the behavior of the offender. Prior to the rape law reform movement, most statutes required that the victim prove nonconsent by physical resistance to the attack. Rape was the only crime in which resistance by the victim had to be proven. Many statutes now focus on the force or threat of force made by the offender rather than the consent of the victim. Laws differ as to whether consent can be used as a defense after charges have been filed.

Linked to the issue of consent is the admissibility of the victim's past sexual history. A history of sexual activity with the offender or with others had been used to show a pattern of behavior that implied consent. Feminist reformers pushed hard for rape shield provisions that would disallow grilling victims about their sexual history. Rape shield laws have been enacted in every state except Utah (Epstein and Langenbahn, 1994), although they vary from state to state in how much and under what circumstances evidence of a victim's previous sexual behavior can be admitted. Some consider rape shield provisions one of the most important aspects of reform to victims, increasing their comfort with prosecution (Goldberg-Ambrose, 1992; Epstein and Langenbahn, 1994). Yet as noted above, there is no evidence that these changes have had an impact on the actual evidence that is allowed in court (Horney and Spohn, 1991).

Other aspects of rape laws that served to call into question the veracity of the victim have also been changed. Most of the laws have dropped the necessity to have corroborating witnesses. Since rape is most often committed by lone offenders in an isolated setting, the need for witnesses made prosecution of rape extremely difficult. Convictions were often also said to be hampered by the requirement of cautionary instructions to the jury, in which the judge told the jury prior to deliberations that they must consider how easy it was to bring false accusations of rape. The use of cautionary instructions has been dropped in most states.

Although national rates of reporting of sexual assaults increased between 1970 and 1980 (Bourque, 1989), research has found only minor effects in some locations on rates of arrest, prosecution, or conviction as a result of legal reforms. The reforms may not have resulted in changes in these rates, because, in some instances, practices were already changing prior to the legal reform (Horney and Spohn, 1991), and in others, the amount of decision-making discretion available to prosecutors and judges maintained previous practices (Loh, 1980; Goldberg-Ambrose, 1992). Other changes in the criminal justice system, as well as social changes during that time, make it difficult to attribute any rate changes in reporting, arrest, prosecution, or conviction to legal reform alone (Goldberg-Ambrose, 1992). Furthermore, Goldberg-Ambrose (1992) reports that some of those most involved in the rape law reform movement identified symbolic and educational effects of reform as the most important consequences of legal change (Nordby, 1980; Bienen, 1983; Chappell, 1984). From that perspective, legal reforms could be thought of as a preventive intervention.

Rape within marriage presents special legal problems. For most of Western history, marital rape was not considered a crime. Its recognition as a crime today is by no means universal and remains controversial, despite evidence that rape within marriage is often repeated and extremely brutal (Browne, 1987; Pagelow, 1988). The marital exemption to rape is a carryover from the days of coverture—when married women had no legal identity separate from their husbands and the marriage vow was considered equivalent to the woman's consent to sexual access. A few states have completely eliminated the marital exemption from their law; others have enacted legislation that makes some rapes within marriage a crime; and in other states court actions have essentially overturned the marital exemption (Russell, 1991). Assessing the effects of changes in marital rape laws may be even more difficult than assessing the effects of the other legal reforms. The National Clearinghouse on Marital and Date Rape compiled statistics on the number of marital rape arrests between 1978 and 1985 and found that 56 percent of the arrests resulted in prosecution and 88 percent of the prosecuted cases resulted in conviction (Russell, 1991). Russell (1991) speculates that this high conviction rate may be attributed to wives only reporting extremely violent cases of marital rape.

The Uniform Crime Reports (Federal Bureau of Investigation, 1993) do not keep track of offender-victim relationships, so it is difficult to ascertain how many marital rapes are reported to police. Twenty-six percent of the rapes and sexual assaults reported on the 1992-1993 National Crime Victimization Survey (Bachman and Saltzman, 1995) were committed by an intimate (i.e., husband, ex-husband, boyfriend, or ex-boyfriend).

Law Enforcement and Prosecution

Institutional changes have taken place both in law enforcement and prosecutors' offices with regard to sexual assaults. Many large city police forces have established specialized sex crime units, while smaller forces may give specialized training to individual investigators (Epstein and Langenbahn, 1994). These specialized units can help ensure that appropriate forensic evidence is collected. Prosecutors' offices also have specialized units that handle sex crimes. Both police and prosecutors may make use of in-house victim advocates or advocates from rape crisis centers to work with victims and serve as a liaison between victims and the legal system.

For cases that go to trial, the jury's preconceived notions about rape may interfere with conviction. Legal reforms excluding cautionary instructions to the jury and limiting the evidence about the victim's sexual history have been instituted, but their effects are not well known and may not be as anticipated. In fact, in one study that played tapes of real rape trials to simulated jurors (reported in Temkin, 1987), the jurors were more likely to convict in a case with a cautionary instruction than in one without. Besides eliminating prejudicial testimony, a more recent tact by prosecutors has been the introduction of expert testimony on rape myth acceptance, and on posttraumatic stress disorder or rape trauma syndrome. While there is a growing amount of legal literature on the admissibility of such testimony in rape trials, no research has actually tested the impact of this testimony on jurors (Goldberg-Ambrose, 1992).

Another aspect of implementing legal sanctions for sexual assault that has received some research attention is the effect of race of both the victim and the offender. LaFree (1989) noted that virtually all research done prior to 1970 found that black defendants receive more serious official sanctions than white defendants, while most research conducted after 1970 found little evidence of discrimination. However, much of the recent research has not examined the entire range of criminal justice processing. LaFree (1989) argues that examining only one or two processing outcomes may show no evidence of discrimination, although the cumulative effect of race over all processes may be considerable. For that reason, LaFree (1989) studied the impact of race of offender and victim from reporting to arrest through prosecution and sentencing. Looking at all forcible sex offenses reported to the Indianapolis police in 1970, 1973, and 1975, LaFree (1989:145) concluded that "black offender-white victim rapes resulted in substantially more serious penalties than other rapes, even controlling for the case characteristics that are most often included in this type of research. Moreover, black intraracial assaults consistently resulted in the least serious punishment for offenders."

Stalking

Stalking has only recently been recognized by the law as a separate crime, and it is a concern in both intimate partner violence and sexual assault. Anecdotal evidence suggests that battered women who attempt to leave their batterers are often stalked by them (e.g., Walker, 1979; Browne, 1987). California passed the first stalking law in 1990. By 1994, 47 other states and the District of Columbia had passed stalking laws, many of them patterned after the California statute (Sohn, 1994). These antistalking laws prohibit a person from following or harassing another person with the intent to cause the victim to fear imminent death or serious bodily injury. Critics of antistalking legislation contend that the laws are overbroadly written and that harassment and other types of threatening behavior were already illegal in most states (Sohn, 1994). Because these laws have so recently been passed, there has not yet been an opportunity to study whether they will make victims of stalking safer or not.

TREATMENT INTERVENTIONS

Intervening with batterers in order to change their behavior emerged as a reaction to frustration among shelter workers who saw women revictimized after returning home to an unchanged male partner or saw the batterer move on to a new victim. Although batterers were being seen in individual and marital therapy, shelter workers and other women's advocates believed a different type of program was needed and began to develop group programs for male batterers in the late 1970s. Programs such as EMERGE in Boston (Adams and McCormick, 1982) and the Duluth model (Pence and Paymar, 1993) have been emulated in many locations (Feazell et al., 1984; Pirog-Good and Stets-Kealey, 1985). As more and more communities began to arrest batterers, mandating them to a group intervention became popular. At the same time as group programs for batterers were expanding, the family therapy model of counseling was also growing. This treatment focused on couples and family counseling efforts with men who abused their partners (Geller and Walsh, 1977-1978; Coleman, 1980).

While court-mandated treatment for batterers may be recommended in lieu of incarceration, treatment of convicted rapists and other sex offenders usually occurs as part of incarceration. Nearly all state correction systems offer some type of counseling or treatment for incarcerated sex offenders, and 19 states have separate facilities for at least some sex offenders (Maguire and Pastore, 1995). Treatments include insight-oriented, cognitive-behavioral, behavioral modification, and pharmacological therapies (Prentky, 1990).

Batterers' Groups

Counseling or educational groups for men who batter have emerged as the most common form of intervention for offenders in the United States (Feazell et al., 1984; Pirog-Good and Stets-Kealy, 1985; Gondolf, 1987; Caesar and Hamberger, 1989; Gondolf, 1995). Group treatment is believed by many to be more appropriate than individual treatment because it expands the social networks of batterers to include other men who are supportive of being nonabusive. It also provides men an opportunity to reinforce their own learning by helping teach others (Edleson and Tolman, 1992). Furthermore, men have reported group support as being one of the most beneficial aspects of treatment (Gondolf, 1985; Tolman, 1990). However, there is a danger that the group may reinforce negative behavior rather than change. In a study of batterers' groups, Tolman (1990) received reports of negative effects from some of the female partners of the men.

Batterers' groups vary in length of time, although most are relatively short term, ranging from 6 to 32 weeks (Eisikovits and Edleson, 1989; Tolman and Bennett, 1990). Programs are generally structured in format and use some variation of cognitive-behavioral or social learning approaches (Tolman and Edleson, 1995; for a more complete discussion of structure of groups, see Edleson and Tolman, 1992). Many programs also include a gendered analysis of battering: that is, battering is viewed as a tool of male control of women in intimate relationships. The focus of the program is as much on changing men's view of their entitlement to control their partners, through whatever means, as it is on stopping the actual physical battering (see, e.g., Pence and Paymar, 1993).

A number of researchers have studied batterers' groups to see how effective they are in stopping physical violence (e.g., Purdy and Nickle, 1981; Edleson et al., 1985; Dutton, 1986; Hamberger and Hastings, 1986; Rosenbaum, 1986; Waldo, 1986; DeMaris and Jackson, 1987; Edleson and Grusznski, 1989; Tolman and Bhosley, 1989; Edleson and Syers, 1990; Palmer et al., 1992; Saunders, 1994). The findings are somewhat positive, but they must be cautiously interpreted due to many methodological shortcomings. Most of the studies did not use control groups, making it impossible to ascribe outcomes to the treatment; sample sizes were frequently small; and attrition in both the programs and the study follow-up periods was high. It is also difficult to compare results across studies because outcomes were measured differently: some studies relied on official records, for example, looking at re-arrest rates; others relied on information reported by the batterers; still others gathered information from the partners of the batterers. The length of the posttreatment follow-up period varied from a few months to several years. Because of these many methodological shortcomings and differences, some analysts have concluded that there is little that one can conclude about the effectiveness of these treatment programs (Hamberger and Hastings, 1993). Others are more optimistic, noting that there are consistent findings that a large proportion of men stop their physically abusive behavior after involvement in a program (Tolman and Edleson, 1995). Studies that relied on partners' reports of physical abuse have found between 53 percent and 85 percent success rates in follow-up periods ranging from 4 to 26 months (Edleson and Tolman, 1992).

There is little information about interventions for batterers who are racial or ethnic minorities. In a recent survey of 142 batterers' programs, the majority did not provide services that targeted minority clients. For example, only 25 percent of the programs provided education and training in minority communities. Even fewer programs incorporated specific program elements designed to encourage minority participation (Williams and Becker, 1994). Anecdotal evidence from programs designed specifically for African American men suggest that they are more successful with that population than other batterers' programs (O.J. Williams, 1992, 1994, 1995). The development and dissemination of culturally relevant programs and policies would benefit from program descriptions and outcome evaluations.

Couples Therapy

The use of couples therapy when there is abuse in a relationship is highly controversial. Many practitioners think that the dynamics of the battering relationship do not lend themselves to joint therapy, especially in court-referred cases (e.g., Dobash and Dobash, 1992; Kaufman, 1992). Most important is the potential of putting the woman in greater danger as a result of the therapy. Those who advocate profeminist approaches to batterers' treatment think that couples therapy, particularly if it focuses on the couple as a system, may allow the batterer to continue to deny responsibility for his violence (Breines and Gordon, 1983; Bograd, 1984).

Little research has been done on the effectiveness of couples therapy in ending violent behavior. Several studies of couples counseling found a reduction or cessation of violence in a sizable proportion of the sample following couples counseling (Taylor, 1984; Neidig et al., 1985; Deschner et al., 1986). However, the samples were small (only 15 couples in one study), the follow-up time was short, and the studies did not specify how violent behavior after treatment was assessed. The last point is particularly important because it has been consistently found that men who batter often report their use of violence to be less frequent and less severe than is reported by their female partners (Szinovacz, 1983; Jouriles and

O'Leary, 1985; Edleson and Brygger, 1986; Bohannon et al., 1995). A recent study comparing couples and single-sex group therapies with couples who had experienced physical aggression—none of it severe—and who wanted to stay together found significant decreases in physical aggression from both therapies a year after therapy ended (O'Leary et al., 1995). Similarly, Harris and colleagues (1988) found no difference in the level of violence or participants' level of psychological well-being between couples who participated in individual couples counseling and those in a group program that consisted of single-sex group sessions followed by couples group sessions. However, participants were four times more likely to drop out of individual couples counseling than the group program. Although there is some evidence that couples therapy may be effective in reducing violence, philosophical disagreements about its use are bound to continue. There is, however, agreement among most practitioners that couples therapy is not appropriate for court-mandated cases or for severely violent men (who are likely to be more violent) (Gondolf, 1995).

Sex Offenders

The question of treatment effectiveness for rapists is the subject of significant controversy. Reviews of treatment outcome studies arrive at different conclusions. An influential paper by Furby et al. (1989) concluded that the methodological problems with most available studies precluded drawing any definitive conclusions. They note that most studies did not carefully describe the treatments, included a mixed group of offenders, and, most importantly, did not have a comparison group of untreated offenders. A recent review had a more optimistic assessment of the available studies, but concluded that even effective programs "do far better with child molesters and exhibitionists than with rapists" (Marshall et al., 1991:481).

The debate about whether the currently available body of

treatment outcome literature is informative on the question of treatment effectiveness revolves around the scientific merit of the studies. It is argued that without formal controlled clinical trials with untreated comparison groups, recidivism rates cannot be attributed to the intervention (Quinsey et al., 1993). But there are moral and ethical constraints—as well as community objections—to withholding treatment from known sex offenders that argue against trying to achieve this standard of scientific rigor. Marshall (1993) contends that it is possible to accumulate knowledge about treatment effectiveness by identifying appropriate comparison groups among those who refuse treatment or for some reason do not receive the specified treatment. He believes that any reduction in recidivism is worthwhile because of the enormous cost of even a single repeat offense to the victim and society.

There is one study that used a random assignment design with control groups that provides specific data on rapists (Marques et al., 1994). The treatment consisted of a comprehensive cognitive behavioral program that used a "relapse prevention" framework, in which offenders are taught to identify situations and emotional states in which they are likely to reoffend and the skills to avoid those situations and deal with the emotional states. Preliminary results for the 59 rapists (as opposed to child molesters) in the study revealed reoffense rates within 5 years of prison release (as measured by rearrest) for sex offenses of 9 percent for the treatment group, 28 percent for the offenders who volunteered but were not assigned to the treatment condition, and 11 percent for the nonvolunteer control group. The rates for other violent offenses were 23 percent for the treatment group, 33 percent for the volunteer controls, and 22 percent for the nonvolunteer controls. It is unfortunate that the total treatment sample includes so few rapists, and therefore, the power necessary for statistical analyses is reduced. It is worth noting that the overall reoffense rates are relatively modest considering current beliefs about the risk for recidivism among rapists. There was one striking finding: of the rapists who had to be removed from the treatment group for seriously disruptive behavior, 100 percent committed a new sex offense. It is possible that offenders with a particularly high risk of reoffending can be identified as those who are too disruptive to participate in treatment programs.

Many questions remain about what treatment for rapists should entail and whether it is a worthwhile endeavor, as opposed to simply imposing long periods of incarceration. Efforts might be useful to identify those who are at highest risk for reoffending and imposing especially long sentences on them. An actuarial method for prediction of future sexual dangerousness has been developed (Quinsey et al., 1995): variables such as prior convictions, deviant sexual interests, and psychopathy have been shown to be associated with increased risk. However, there are major philosophical questions involved in sentencing on the basis of future predicted behavior.

CONCLUSIONS AND RECOMMENDATIONS

There are few good evaluations of preventive or treatment interventions for either victims or perpetrators of violence against women. Existing evaluations are difficult to compare because different outcomes have been measured in different ways and at different times. One serious problem with studies of interventions is selecting and operationally defining outcomes to measure. For example, is the goal of a batterers' treatment program to reduce or completely stop batterers' violent behavior? Should prevention programs measure reduction in victimization rates or reduction in perpetration rates? Should services for battered women consider improvement in self-esteem, separation from the batterer, or physical safety as the outcome? Should treatment of rapists measure sexual arousal or behavior outside the laboratory as an outcome? At what intervals following the completion of the program should measurements be made? Are there unintended negative outcomes from prevention or treatment interventions? Close collaboration between researchers and practitioners is necessary to carefully specify the basic assumptions underlying the intervention and to determine what outcomes constitute success.

> **Recommendation: Evaluations of preventive and treatment intervention efforts must clearly define the outcomes expected from the intervention. These outcome measures should derive from an explicit theory underlying each intervention. Defining outcomes requires close collaboration between researchers and service providers.**

Preventive Interventions

School-based programs to prevent date rape and intimate partner violence, as well as programs on conflict resolution and general violence prevention, have become popular in recent years. However, these programs have seldom been evaluated, and the evaluations that have been done usually look only at short-term attitudinal change. Their longer term impact on behavior, arguably what these programs are trying to effect, remains unknown. In light of studies that have detected negative outcomes with some program participants, a better understanding of long-term outcomes and differential effects of preventive efforts is needed.

Early childhood predictors have been identified for violence in adolescence and adulthood as well as for other undesirable behavior (e.g. substance abuse, teenage pregnancy). Some of the predictors that have been identified include impaired relationships with parents, witnessing violence, experiencing physical abuse and neglect, absence of prosocial role models, and early learning and behavior problems. It is possible that sexual and intimate partner violence have common precursors with other forms of violent and dysfunctional or undesirable behavior. Except for the few prevention programs targeted at preventing dating violence, most youth violence prevention programs have ignored the prevention of intimate partner and sexual violence. Inclusion of the consideration of violence against women in these studies would greatly increase understanding of possible links between various types of violent behavior and might lead to better designed prevention programs.

> **Recommendation: Programs designed to prevent sexual and intimate partner violence should be subject to rigorous evaluation of both short- and long-term effects. Programs designed to prevent delinquency, substance abuse, teenage pregnancy, gang involvement, or general violence (including conflict mediation programs) should include evaluation of risk factors for and prevention of intimate and sexual violence. In addition, studies of at-risk children and adolescents should include an examination of the relationship of risk factors, such as poverty, childhood victimization, and brain injury, to outcomes of sexual and intimate partner violence.**

Interventions with Victims

Services for victims of rape and domestic violence are available in many communities. Anecdotal evidence and the few evaluation studies that have been done seem to indicate that the services are helpful to the women who use them. Yet many women do not use those services. Research is needed to determine whether those women are unaware of the services; if the services offered fail to meet their needs; if they seek help from systems, either formal or informal, other than those specifically designed for victims of violence against women; if they do not want or need services; or if other factors play a part in their underutilitzation or nonutilization of services. Special attention should be paid to whether there are systematic differences in the types of services sought by different subpopulations of women, and, if so, the implications of those differences for providing services. A better understanding of both the effectiveness of current services and the service needs that remain unmet could lead to better program designs. Furthermore, studying women who do not seek services may yield information on factors that affect resiliency and obviate the need for services. An understanding of the social, economic, and institutional barriers that may prevent women from seeking services is important to designing these alternatives. For example, services might be made available in primary health care, community clinics, or educational facilities. In spite of the proliferation of training and screening protocols, particularly for professionals in medical settings, violent victimization is frequently overlooked. The effectiveness of training programs needs to be assessed to determine the training models that best equip professionals to identify and assist victims.

Recommendation: Studies that describe current services for victims of violence and evaluate their effectiveness are needed. Studies to investigate the factors associated with victims' service-seeking behavior, including delaying seeking of services or not seeking services at all, are also needed. These studies should describe and evaluate innovative or alternative approaches or settings for identifying and providing services to victims of violence against women.

Interventions with Offenders

Interventions with sex offenders and batterers consist of a criminal justice response or specialized social service treatment programs for certain offenders, or both. Information is needed to determine the relative effectiveness of various interventions and to develop a means of matching offenders to interventions. Special attention should be paid to cultural and ethnic differences that may have a bearing on the effectiveness of interventions. Studies should not overlook possible informal surveillance and control mechanisms that may work independently or in conjunction with more formal controls to deter offenders from repeating their violent behavior. Efforts are also needed to find effective interventions for the large subset of offenders for whom current approaches are ineffective.

The panel considers court-mandated programs for batterers to be ripe for randomized, controlled outcome studies. Such programs are gaining in number around the country. Criminal justice personnel, judges, and victims all seem to find mandated batterers' programs an attractive option. As these mandated programs proliferate, it is important to understand what features—including other community resources and concomitant sanctions, as well as program philosophy, structure, and length—make them effective, and for whom.

> **Recommendation: Randomized, controlled outcome studies are needed to identify the program and community features that account for the effectiveness of legal or social service interventions with various groups of offenders.**

Criminal Justice System

The crimes of rape and battery by intimate partners have historically been handled and perceived differently than other person-to-person crimes. Legal reforms have been proposed and implemented to treat sexual assault and intimate partner violence similarly to other crimes, but little is known about how these reforms have affected actual practices or what differences, if any, they have made for victims. For example, many changes have been made in rape laws and rape trial procedures, but little is known about the impact of those changes on investigation, prosecutorial decision making, or jury behavior. Similarly, the use of expert witnesses on the results of trauma (e.g., rape trauma syndrome, posttraumatic stress syndrome, and battered woman's syndrome) is becoming more widespread, but few studies have been done on the effects of such testimony on trial outcome. More broadly, there is little information on the way in which reforms interact with people and practices within the systems. The process by which reforms are implemented, or not implemented, may well be as important as the reforms themselves.

Recommendation: Studies are needed that examine discretionary processes in the criminal and civil justice systems, including implementation of new laws and reforms, charging and prosecutorial decision making, jury decision making, and judicial decision making. Legal research, which supplies the theoretical basis behind legal interpretations and reforms, is also needed.

NOTES

1. The advocates used in this study were trained undergraduates; some researchers and practitioners speculate that the impact of advocacy may have been greater if professional advocates had been used.

2. A research grant from the National Institute of Mental Health supported the 1975 National Survey on Family Violence (Straus et al., 1980). The Law Enforcement Assistance Administration (LEAA) funded local criminal justice initiatives on behalf of victims during the 1970s. LEAA established a Family Violence Program to fund demonstration and evaluation programs in 1978 (see Fagan et al., 1984). The interests, knowledge, and concerns of victim advocates, researchers, and policy makers were heard in a 1978 consultation sponsored by the U.S. Commission on Civil Rights and later that year in hearings on battering before a subcommittee of the U.S. Senate Committee on Human Resources. See Schechter (1982) for a critical discussion of these developments.

3. Mandatory arrest means that an officer must arrest if he or she finds probable cause that a crime was committed; a presumptive arrest policy allows the officer discretion, calling for arrest unless the officer believes that circumstances dictate some alternative.

5

Research Infrastructure

Various disciplines have contributed to the development of research on violence against women, including psychology, psychiatry, medicine, nursing, public health, social work, statistics, epidemiology, sociology, ethnography, anthropology, social history, criminology, and law. Each discipline brings different theoretical models, databases, instrumentation, and problem definitions to its work. As a result, it is often extremely difficult to generalize from clusters of studies or to build on earlier work.

With the passage of the Violence Against Women Act of 1994 (Title IV of P.L. 103-322), the federal government initiated a broad set of programs focused on violence against women, many of which will be administered by law enforcement, prosecution, and victim services organizations. Hotline services, victim advocate programs, and shelter resources represent important community-based programs that can respond to the immediate needs of women in crisis as a result of violence. However, these same programs are often not equipped to deal effectively with research knowledge in the development of their services, and, conversely, their collective experiences in dealing with women affected or threatened by violence are often not accessible or used by the researchers.

TRAINING RESEARCHERS AND PRACTITIONERS

The community of researchers whose work focuses on understanding, controlling, or preventing violence against women is extremely small. Although this community has developed some networks in communicating research findings of common interest across disciplines, it lacks the resources or opportunities to integrate this research into other fields of study and practice. Furthermore, this field of research is characterized by the absence of clear conceptual models, large-scale data bases, longitudinal research, and reliable instrumentation. Investigators have difficulty obtaining funding because their research proposals often compete against those from more established fields that can build on an infrastructure developed through decades of prior research activity. Investigators may also lack opportunities to learn from relevant research in areas that can enrich the development of research on violence, such as deterrence theory in criminal behavior, the study of community-based organizational behavior, the effectiveness of formal and informal controls in governing individual and group behavior, research on the use of community services, adolescent health, the cultural context of coercion and power, and program evaluation, particularly models of community responses that have been developed in such fields as substance abuse prevention (see, e.g., Kaftarian and Hansen, 1994).

At the same time, there is increasing need for researchers who understand violence against women and can put that understanding to work with practitioners to improve program design and evaluation. In these days of budget cutbacks, programs will increasingly be called on to show evidence of their effectiveness through systematic evaluation. Program evaluation studies of treatment and prevention services in this field will require improved efforts to design outcome studies that target violence reduction as a specific measure of the effectiveness of the program under review. Such studies will require careful design and attention to a range of concerns that are often associated with other community-based program evaluation studies, including the theoretical strength of the selected program, fidelity of implementation of the particular activity that is under review, the length of follow-up, the availability of a matched control group, and the size of the sample. Such studies will require researchers and practitioners who are able and willing to work together to achieve better evaluation studies that can inform and improve interventions.

There are also training needs among related professionals who are in positions to identify women victims of violence. For example, a broad set of initiatives has been developed to improve the diagnostic skills of emergency room health personnel, obstetric-gynecologist physicians, and primary care practitioners in detecting and responding effectively to battered women and to sexually assaulted women. However, many mental health and health care professionals who are responsible for the treatment of women for substance abuse, mental health disorders, or sexually transmitted diseases have not received the same type of educational effort designed to highlight the importance of identifying the role of violent trauma in the course of complex health behaviors. Other neglected health care fields are the areas of pediatrics, adolescent medicine, sports medicine, and the military and veterans' health care systems, which often have very broad access to young men but which virtually ignore any attempt to identify risk factors for violent behavior in the course of primary care treatment. All too often, the result in health care is a "field" that sees fragmented aspects of physical and mental health problems that share common risk factors and common origins but lacks a means of connecting them and the presenting symptoms to a recommended course of treatment. The effort to integrate research on violence against women into the training and certification requirements for a wide community of health professionals thus confronts a tremendous challenge that requires constructive approaches in the decade ahead. One promising proposal is for the inclusion of information on many forms of violence, including battering and sexual assault, in training, continuing education, and certification requirements for a variety of professions, such as law, law enforcement, nursing, social work, and education (Minnesota Higher Education Center Against Violence and Abuse, 1995).

A topic that is often missing in the training of both researchers and practitioners is information on diverse population groups—at the same time that both researchers and practitioners are frequently exhorted to be sensitive to cultural differences and to be culturally competent. These concepts were well described by the Institute of Medicine's Committee on Reducing Mental Disorders (Mrazek and Haggerty, 1994:391-392):

> Cultural sensitivity is the awareness of a body of important information relevant to the population(s) of interest, which should inform the entire research process, from defining the sampling frame, through negotiating access, to actual intervention and dissemination of results. Such sensitivity can be, and typically is, learned through formal, didactic means and by familiarity with the rapidly growing literatures. It is a necessary but insufficient condition for cultural competence. Cultural competence is achieved through personal experience, either closely supervised practice or actual immersion in the field, which leads to acquisition and mastery of the skills needed to fit interventions to context.

There is little information characterizing the experience of violence among racial and ethnic minority women or among women who are homeless, poor, substance abusers, recent immigrants, migrants, disabled, or lesbian. It is in these areas, where violence is often thought to be more prevalent because of the nature of the dependency of women and their social isolation, that researchers are most poorly equipped to understand the forms, nature, or scope of gender-specific violent behavior. Services targeted for these populations are also often lacking.

Training is needed to prepare researchers and practitioners to meet the challenges of culturally competent research and interventions, by exposing them to the relevant literature, teaching qualitative research techniques as well as quantitative ones, and providing opportunities to interact with the communities they are studying or serving. Training more minority researchers and service providers may also be beneficial in broadening research and intervention contexts to include underserved and understudied populations.

As in other fields for which resources are insufficient to meet demand for services, practitioners may see researchers as competitors for scarce funds. Research is also seen by some practitioners as irrelevant to providing services. Researchers, for their part, may ignore the experiential knowledge base of those who have worked with battered women or rape victims or fail to make their findings accessible to the practitioner community. Although many individual researchers have established contacts and collaborations with practitioners, this is a time-intensive task that is not necessarily supported by current research infrastructure and funding mechanisms. Practitioners who want input from researchers or technical assistance in planning and evaluating programs have to spend scarce time and resources locating researchers to help them.

FUNDING

The issue of violence against women has received increased attention at the federal level in recent years, accompanied by targeted funding for programs and research. Research funding is based primarily in three agencies: the National Institute of Justice (NIJ) of the U.S. Department of Justice, and the Centers for Disease Control and Prevention

(CDC) and the National Institutes of Health (NIH) of the U.S. Department of Health and Human Services (HHS). A variety of other federal agencies have also supported individual studies on violence against women, including HHS's Administration for Children and Families (ACF), the U.S. Department of Labor, and the U.S. Department of Education.

Despite some efforts in the past 2 years to coordinate activities relating to violence, however, the funding remains fragmentary, and no single agency is responsible for determining the overall level of funding for research (or programs). As a consequence, it is extremely difficult to determine how much money the federal government is currently investing in violence against women research. It is even difficult to locate information on funded projects or the results of funded research. Without such information, it is difficult to evaluate the scope and emphasis of the federal effort, to improve dissemination of research findings, and to identify research gaps. The panel did not have the resources within its 1-year study to identify or comprehensively review all federal research; rather, it could only catalog some of the larger areas of research activity.

In fiscal 1994, $7.3 million was appropriated to the CDC to undertake a program to prevent violence against women (Centers for Disease Control and Prevention, 1995). Activities have been developed to meet five broad goals: describing and tracking the problem, increasing knowledge of causes and consequences, demonstrating and evaluating ways to prevent violence against women, supporting a national communications effort, and fostering a nationwide network of prevention and support services. The CDC's National Center for Injury Prevention and Control is overseeing this effort and is currently spending about $1.8 million a year in extramural research efforts.

Over the past 4 years, NIJ has awarded more than $1 million annually to research and evaluation projects on family violence (National Institute of Justice, 1995), which includes child abuse, battering, and elder abuse. NIJ has indicated that it plans to allocate a percentage of its program funds under the Violence Against Women Act for evaluation research, but the nature of this activity has not yet been defined.

In 1993 the Administration for Children and Families awarded funding to establish the national Domestic Violence Resource Network, composed of the National Resource Center on Domestic Violence, the Battered Women's Justice Project, the Health Resource Center on Domestic Violence, and the Resource Center on Child Protection and Custody. The members of the Resource Network collect information and support services for battered women and their children. The resource centers provide important distribution points for program-related information, but their efforts do not have a primary focus on research studies or on tracking what may be relevant findings from studies in this field.

Other federal agencies have also provided funding for research on violence against women, particularly two NIH institutes. In fiscal 1994, the National Institute of Mental Health (NIMH) spent about $2.5 million on physical and sexual violence studies and the National Institute on Alcohol Abuse and Alcoholism (NIAAA) spent about $314,000 on studies dealing with sexual assault and alcohol and battering and alcohol.

At present there are no state research centers focused primarily on violence against women. However, individual training projects in the area of prosecution and law enforcement provide important regional and national resources that reveal key characteristics of law enforcement and judicial policy and process that may impede or contribute to the reduction of violence against women.

No private foundations have established violence against women as a primary area of programmatic emphasis, but several foundations are developing research programs in various aspects of family and community violence that have implications for the field. The Family Violence Prevention Fund, for example, which is funded by the California Wellness Foundation and other private foundations, has established a major initiative designed to foster reform in health care practices in the treatment and prevention of violence against women. The Conrad N. Hilton Foundation has recently made domestic violence one of its four funding areas.

A number of private foundations and corporations have supported services for victimized women. For example, the Domestic Violence Prevention Project in New York City received initial funding from the Robert Sterling Clark Foundation, the New York Community Trust, the Norman Foundation, and the Conrad N. Hilton Foundation, and the Ford Foundation supported evaluation of the project. Other foundations are beginning to explore the issue of violence against women within the context of improving women's health. The Commonwealth Fund, for example, is sponsoring the Women's Health Initiative, which organized a symposium on violence against women, held in New York City in September 1995, to examine the implications of violent behavior for the health outcomes of women.

CONCLUSIONS AND RECOMMENDATIONS

Research on violence against women will be strengthened by a research infrastructure that supports interdisciplinary efforts and helps to integrate those efforts into service programs and institutional policies, especially in the area of preventive intervention. Key areas for improving research infrastructure are coordination and leadership at the federal level and improving research capacity and strengthening ties between researchers and practitioners.

Government Coordination and Leadership

At the national level, three major agencies provide most of the research funding for violence against women—the Centers for Disease Control and Prevention, the National Institute of Justice, and the National Institutes of Health—with some funding from other agencies. In addition, many other agencies, including the National Science Foundation and the Department of Education, have programs that could contribute to the development of research on violence against women. Special efforts are needed to strengthen the role of these agencies in a collaborative effort at the national level. A mechanism for information sharing, interdisciplinary research development, research collaboration, and collaborative dissemination across agencies is needed. The panel has taken note of on-going collaborative efforts and applauds the agencies for them. Added efforts are needed to ensure the continuation of these collaborations and bring in agencies that are not yet part of the collaboration.

Providing effective leadership requires not only collaboration among agencies, but also a coordination of effort. Coordination might best be achieved through the designation of a lead agency on violence against women. Current government efforts have centered around criminal justice interventions, such as the establishment of the Office on Violence Against Women at the U.S. Department of Justice and NIJ's decision to set aside a proportion of its Violence Against Women Act funds for research in this field. These steps should help ensure a strong criminal justice system involvement in violence against women programs and research. However, the focus of research efforts must go beyond criminal justice.

The panel believes that in order to significantly reduce the amount of violence against women in the United States the focus must be on prevention. This suggests that an agency with more interdisciplinary, prevention-oriented experience than NIJ coordinate the federal research effort on violence against women. The panel recognizes that prevention is a long-term strategy—that research must continue on criminal justice interventions with individual perpetrators of violence against women and on social service, health, and mental health interventions for victims—but it should guide the overall effort in this field.

Recommendation: The panel recommends that government agencies develop a coordinated strategy to strengthen the creation of a research base that is focused on prevention of violence against women and interventions for offenders and victims.

One way to achieve this goal would be the formation of a federal Task Force on Research on Violence Against Women with representation from all relevant agencies and a chair that rotates between the U.S. Department of Justice and the U.S. Department of Health and Human Services. Coordination of government-supported research in the field of violence against women could be further improved through the designation of a lead agency to track all federal research and expenditures on violence against women and identify research gaps. Should a lead agency be designated, the panel believes that agency should be the Centers for Disease Control and Prevention because of CDC's record of experience with interdisciplinary and prevention research.

Improving Research Capacity and Strengthening Research-Provider Collaboration

In many fields, research centers have been successful in developing innovative, interdisciplinary research. Examples of such efforts include the CDC-funded Injury Control Research Centers, the NIMH-funded Minority Mental Health Research Centers, the Children's Safety Network funded by the Maternal and Child Health Bureau, and the NIMH-funded Preventive Intervention Research Centers (PIRC). Research centers are usually funded for extended periods of time, allowing for the development of excellent in-depth theoretical, methodological, and applied research focused on a specific topic. The PIRC model may be particularly applicable to issues related to violence against women: its funding mechanism allows for a combination of basic, intervention, and methodological studies that can inform each other. This combination led to an integration of careful scientific theory and process into all phases of design, testing, and dissemination of preventive interventions (Koretz, 1991). Research emanating from the PIRCs has been at the forefront of efforts to move preventive intervention research away from simple outcome assessments of atheoretical intervention strategies toward experimental tests of population-based, theoretically derived models. This development has led to a greater understanding of causal mechanisms and processes of the various conditions that are the focus of individual PIRCs and to innovative methodologies for overcoming the many challenges of doing field experimentation.

Research centers can also serve as a potent mechanism for research and practitioner collaboration and for training. The flexibility inherent in the funding for many research centers allows for the creation and evaluation of demonstration service delivery projects that require the talents and skills of both practitioners and researchers and also provide opportunities for training young researchers and practitioners. Research centers that include a technical assistance component can serve as a resource for service delivery programs in surrounding communities, helping them to incorporate research findings into their programs and helping them design and carry out program evaluations. The history of past research endeavors leads the panel to question whether topics relating to women's experiences of violence would receive adequate attention without resources earmarked specifically for them.

Recommendation: The panel recommends that a minimum of three to four research centers be established within academic or other appropriate settings to support the development of studies and training programs focused on violence against women, to provide mechanisms for collaboration between researchers and practitioners and technical assistance for integrating research into service provision.

The panel believes that research centers specifically devoted to violence against women are important to expanding and improving the knowledge base. The centers could be organized as regional centers or each could have a particular focus. The experience of PIRCs and the Injury Control Research Centers with focused centers leads the panel to prefer that model over a regional model. The centers could be organized around research areas such as the epidemiology and measurement of violence against women, causes and risk factors for violence against women, and preventive and treatment intervention evaluation research. Or centers could be organized around such topics as violence against women in minority and underserved populations, alcohol and drug abuse in violence against women, violence against women in the media, and violence against rural women.

The purpose of the technical assistance aspect of the centers is to encourage state agencies and community-based and other service providers to use theoretical models and research tools and instruments in the design of their service interventions and program evaluation. Service providers are increasingly being called on by funders to evaluate their programs. Providers also have contact with large numbers of victims and offenders and offer unique opportunities for collecting data to better understand violence against women. Yet most service providers lack the technical expertise to plan and carry out research. The technical assistance function of the centers would provide a source of information to improve service providers' ability to collect data and evaluate program effectiveness. Furthermore, dissemination is an inherent part of research, yet all too often research findings never reach the service providers. Technical assistance from the centers would also help to make research findings accessible to service providers; could support technical training programs for service provider agency personnel; and could possibly provide seed money for service providers to conduct small-scale case studies or descriptive reviews of selected program interventions.[1]

The research centers would contribute to the field by incorporating interdisciplinary areas of knowledge; fostering exchanges between and among sciences and the humanities in the development of theory, measurement, social constructs, and policy recommendations; and assisting service providers to develop and carry out well-designed program evaluations. More specifically, the role of the Violence Against Women Research Centers would include the following:

- to foster a dialogue among the disciplines about the nature of violence against women and its relationship to other forms of violence and injury and to develop a conceptual framework that could assess the development of this field;
- to stimulate creative approaches in encouraging service providers' collaboration with researchers on the design and evaluation of program interventions;
- to foster collaborative research efforts among researchers from different disciplines and institutions and between research institutions and service providers;
- to develop training programs for young investigators and to provide curriculum materials to other training institutions;
- to encourage the training of minority researchers;
- to provide a national focus for public forums designed to disseminate research knowledge about violence against women; and
- to provide technical assistance to service providers.

The problem of violence against women in the United States will not be solved in the short term or without concentrated attention. Well-organized research will be critical to and will contribute to the long-term goal of preventing and ameliorating the effects of violence against women.

NOTE

1. It should be noted that these centers would not duplicate the services of the National Resource Center on Domestic Violence, whose focus is not research. These new Violence Against Women Research Centers and their technical assistance functions would cover issues of rape and sexual assault as well as domestic violence and would complement the efforts of the National Resource Center on Domestic Violence.

References

Abbey, A.
  1991 Misperceptions as an antecedent of acquaintance rape: A conse-
        quence of ambiguity in communication between men and women.
        Pp. 96-112 in A. Parrot and L. Bechhofer, eds., *Acquaintance Rape:*
        The Hidden Crime. New York: Wiley.
Abbey, A., L.T. Ross, and D. McDuffie
  1995 Alcohol's role in sexual assault. In R.R. Watson, ed., *Drug and*
        Alcohol Abuse Reviews, Vol. 5: Addictive Behaviors in Women.
        Totowa, N.J.: Humana Press.
Abbott, J., R. Johnson, J. Koziol-McLain, and S.R. Lowenstein
  1995 Domestic violence against women: Incidence and prevalence in
        an emergency room population. *Journal of the American Medical*
        Association 273(22):1763-1767.
Abel, G.G., J.L. Rouleau, and J. Cunningham-Rathner
  1986 Sexually aggressive behavior. In W.J. Curran, A.L. McGarry, and
        S.A. Shah, eds., *Forensic Psychiatry and Psychology: Perspectives*
        and Standards for Interdisciplinary Practice. Philadelphia: F.A.
        Davis.
Adams, D.
  1988 Treatment models of men who batter: A profeminist analysis.
        Pp. 176-200 in K. Yllö and M. Bograd, eds., *Feminist Perspectives*
        on Wife Abuse. Beverly Hills, Calif.: Sage.
Adams, D.C., and A.J. McCormick
  1982 Men unlearning violence: A group approach based on the collec-

tive model. Pp. 170-179 in M. Roy, ed., *The Abusive Partner.*
New York: Van Nostrand Reinhold.

American Educational Research Association, American Psychological Association, and National Council on Measurement in Education
1995   *Standards in Educational and Psychological Testing.* Washington, D.C.: American Psychological Assocation.

American Medical Association
1992   *Diagnostic and Treatment Guidelines on Domestic Violence.* Chicago, Ill.: American Medical Association.

American Psychiatric Association
1994   *Diagnostic and Statistical Manual of Mental Disorders,* 4th ed. (DSM-IV). Washington, D.C.: Author.

Archer, J.
1991   The influence of testosterone on human aggression. *British Journal of Psychology* 82:1-28.

Asberg, M., P. Thoren, and L. Traskman
1976   Serotonin depression: A biochemical subgroup within the affective disorders? *Science* 191:478-480.

Avery-Leaf, S., A. Cano, M. Cascardi, and K.D. O'Leary
1995   Assessing Attitude and Behavioral Change after Dating Violence Intervention Programs. Paper presented at the 4th International Family Violence Research Conference, Durham, New Hampshire, July 21-24. Department of Psychology, State University of New York at Stony Brook.

Bachman, R.
1994   *Violence Against Women: A National Crime Victimization Survey Report.* NCJ-145325. Washington, D.C.: Bureau of Justice Statistics, U.S. Department of Justice.

Bachman, R., and A.L. Coker
1995   Police involvement in domestic violence: The interactive effects of victim injury, offenders's history of violence, and race. *Violence and Victims* 10(2):91-106.

Bachman, R., and L.E. Saltzman
1995   *Violence Against Women: Estimates from the Redesigned Survey.* NCJ-154348. Washington, D.C.: Bureau of Justice Statistics, U.S. Department of Justice.

Baker, K., N. Cahn, and S.J. Sands
1989   *Report on District of Columbia Police Response to Domestic Violence.* Joint project of the D.C. Coalition Against Domestic Violence and the Women's Law and Public Policy Fellowship Program at Georgetown University Law Center. Washington, D.C.: D.C. Coalition Against Domestic Violence.

Baker, T.C., A.W. Burgess, E. Brickman, and R.C. Davis
1990   Rape victims' concerns about possible exposure to HIV infection. *Journal of Interpersonal Violence* 5:49-60.

Bard, M., and D. Sangrey
1986 The Crime Victims' Book. 2nd edition. New York: Brunner/ Mazel.
Barnett, O., and L.K. Hamberger
1992 The assessment of maritally violent men on the California Psychological Inventory. Violence and Victims 7:15-22.
Bart, P.B.
1981 A study of women who both were raped and avoided rape. Journal of Social Issues 37:123-136.
Bart, P.B., R.L. Blumberg, T.Tombs, and F. Behan
1975 The Cross-Societal Study of Rape: Some Methodological Problems and Results. Paper presented at the Groves Conference International Workshop on Changing Sex Roles in Family and Society, Dubrovnik, Yugoslavia.
Bassuk, E., and L. Rosenberg
1988 Why does family homelessness occur? A case-control study. American Journal of Public Health 78(7):783-787.
Bastian, L.
1995 Criminal victimization 1993. Bureau of Justice Statistics Bulletin NCJ-151658, May 1995. Washington, D.C.: Bureau of Justice Statistics, U.S. Department of Justice.
Beebe, D.K.
1991 Emergency management of the adult female rape victim. American Family Physician 43:2041-2046.
Belnap, J.
1989 The sexual victimization of unmarried women by nonrelative acquaintances. Pp. 205-218 in M.A. Pirog-Good and J.E. Stets, eds., Violence in Dating Relationships: Emerging Issues. New York: Praeger.
Berenson, A., N. Stiglich, G. Wilkinson, and G. Anderson
1991 Drug abuse and other risk factors for physical abuse in pregnancy among white non-Hispanic, black, and Hispanic women. American Journal of Obstetrics and Gynecology 164:491-499.
Berk, R.A., P.J. Newton, and S.F. Berk.
1986 What a difference a day makes: An empirical study of the impact of shelters for battered women. Journal of Marriage and the Family 48:431-490.
Berk, R.A., A. Campbell, R. Klap, and B. Western
1992 A Bayesian analysis of the Colorado Springs spouse abuse experiment. Journal of Criminal Law and Criminology 83:170-200.
Berkowitz, A.
1992 College men as perpetrators of acquaintance rape and sexual assault: A review of recent research. Journal of the American College Health Association 40:175-181.
Bienen, L.
1980 Rape III—National developments in rape reform legislation. Women's Rights Law Reporter 6(3):171-213.

1983 Rape reform legislation in the United States: A look at some practice effects. *Victimology* 8:139-151.

Blumstein, A., J. Cohen, and D. Nagin, eds.
1978 *Deterrence and Incapacitation: Estimating the Effects of Criminal Sanctions on Crime Rates.* Panel on Research on Deterrent and Incapacitative Effects, Committee on Research on Law Enforcement and Criminal Justice. Washington, D.C.: National Academy of Sciences.

Bograd, M.
1984 Family systems approaches to wife battering: A feminist critique. *American Journal of Orthopsychiatry* 54:558-568.

Bohannon, J.R., D.A. Dosser, and S.E. Lindley
1995 Using couple data to determine domestic violence rates: An attempt to replicate previous work. *Violence and Victims* 10(2):133-141.

Bohman, M., C.R. Cloninger, S. Sigvardsson, and A.L. von Knorring
1982 Predisposition to petty criminality in Swedish adoptees: I. Genetic and environmental heterogeneity. *Archives of General Psychiatry* 39:1233-1241.

Boney-McCoy, S., and D. Finkelhor
1995 Psychosocial sequelae of violent victimization in a national youth sample. *Journal of Consulting and Clinical Psychology* 63(5):726-736.

Bourque, L.
1989 *Defining Rape.* Durham, N.C.: Duke University Press.

Bowker, L.
1979 The criminal victimization of women. *Victimology* 4:371-384.

Boychuk, M.K.
1994 Are stalking laws unconstitutionally vague or overbroad? *Northwestern University Law Review* 88(2):769-802

Brain, P.F.
1994 Hormonal aspects of aggression and violence. Pp. 173-244 in A.J. Reiss, K.A. Miczek, and J.A. Roth, eds., *Understanding and Preventing Violence: Volume 2, Biobehavioral Influences.* Washington, D.C.: National Academy Press.

Breines, W., and L. Gordon
1983 The new scholarship on family violence. *Signs* 8:490-531.

Brickman, J., and J. Briere
1984 Incidence of rape and sexual assault in an urban Canadian population. *International Journal of Women's Studies* 7:195-206.

Bridges, G., and J.G. Weis
1989 Measuring violent behavior: Effects of study design on reported correlates of violence. In N.A. Weiner and M.E. Wolfgang, eds., *Violent Crime, Violent Criminals.* Newbury Park, Calif.: Sage Publications.

Briere, J.N.
  1992 *Child Abuse Trauma: Theory and Treatment of the Lasting Ef-
         fects.* Newbury Park, Calif.: Sage Publications.
Briere, J., N.M. Malamuth, and J.V.P. Check
  1985 Sexuality and rape-supportive beliefs. *International Journal of
         Women's Studies* 8:396-403.
Brodyaga, L., M. Gates, S. Singer, M. Tucker, and R. White
  1975 *Rape and Its Victims: A Report for Citizens, Health Facilities,
         and Criminal Justice Agencies.* Washington, D.C.: National In-
         stitute of Law Enforcement and Criminal Justice.
Broude, G.J., and S.J. Green
  1976 Cross-cultural codes on twenty sexual attitudes and practices.
         Ethnology 15(4):409-430.
Brown, G.L., F.K. Goodwin, J.C. Ballenger, P.F. Goyer, and L.F. Major
  1979 Aggression in humans correlates with cerebrospinal fluid amine
         metabolites. *Psychiatry Research* 1:131-139.
Brown, J.
  1995 Documenting Change in Battered Women: A Search for Structure
         and Complexity. Paper presented at the 4th International Family
         Violence Research Conference, Durham, New Hampshire, July 21-
         24. Family Violence Research Program, University of Rhode Is-
         land.
Brown, L.S., and M.P.P. Root, eds.
  1990 *Diversity and Complexity in Feminist Therapy.* New York:
         Harrington Park Press.
Browne, A.
  1987 *When Battered Women Kill.* New York: The Free Press.
  1992 Violence against women: Relevance for medical practitioners.
         Journal of the American Medical Association 267:3184-3189.
  1993 Violence against women by male partners: Prevalence, incidence,
         and policy implications. *American Psychologist* 48:1077-1087.
Browne, A., and D.G. Dutton
  1990 Escape from violence: Risks and alternatives for abused women—
         what do we currently know? Pp. 65-91 in R. Roesch, D. G. Dutton,
         and V. F. Sacco, eds., *Family Violence: Perspectives on Treat-
         ment, Research, and Policy.* Burnaby, British Columbia, Canada:
         British Columbia Institute on Family Violence.
Browne, A., and K.R. Williams
  1989 Exploring the effect of resource availability and the likelihood of
         female-perpetrated homicides. *Law and Society Review* 23:75-94.
  1993 Gender, intimacy, and lethal violence: Trends from 1976 through
         1987. *Gender and Society* 7:78-98.
Brownmiller, S.
  1975 *Against Our Will: Men, Women and Rape.* New York: Bantam
         Books.

Bruynooghe, R., and others
1989 Study of physical and sexual violence against Belgian women. Département des Sciences Humaines et Sociales, Limburgs Universitair Centrum, Belgium. As cited in Ada Garcia, *Sexual Violence Against Women: Contribution to a Strategy for Countering the Various Forms of Such Violence in the Council of Europe Member States.* European Committee for Equality between Women and Men, Strasbourg, France, 1991.

Bryer, J.B., B.A. Nelson, J.B. Miller, and P.A. Krol
1987 Childhood sexual and physical abuse as factors in adult psychiatric illness. *American Journal of Psychiatry* 144(11):1426-1430.

Brygger, M.P., and J.L. Edleson
1987 The Domestic Abuse Project: A multisystems intervention in woman battering. *Journal of Interpersonal Violence* 2(3): 324-336.

Bullock, L., and J. McFarlane
1989 The birthweight/battering connection. *Journal of Nursing* 89:1153-1155.

Bureau of Justice Statistics
1994 Selected findings: Violence between intimates. NCJ-149259. Washington, D.C.: U.S. Department of Justice.

Bureau of National Affairs
1990 *Violence and stress: The work/family connection.* Special report #32. Washington, D.C.: Bureau of National Affairs.

Burge, S.K.
1989 Violence against women as a health care issue. *Family Medicine* 21:368-373.

Burgess, A.W., and L.L. Holmstrom
1974 Rape trauma syndrome. *American Journal of Psychiatry* 131:413-418.
1979 Rape: Sexual disruption and recovery. *American Journal of Orthopsychiatry* 49:648-657.

Burnam, M.A., J.A. Stein, J.M. Golding, J.M. Siegel, S.B. Sorenson, A.B. Forsythe, and C.A. Telles
1988 Sexual assault and mental disorders in a community population. *Journal of Consulting and Clinical Psychology* 56:843-850.

Burt, M.R.
1980 Cultural myths and supports for rape. *Journal of Personality and Social Psychology* 38(2):217-230.

Burt, M.R., J. Gornick, and K. Pittman
1984 *Feminism and Rape Crisis Centers.* Washington, D.C.: The Urban Institute.

Buzawa, E.S., and C.G. Buzawa
1990 *Domestic Violence: The Criminal Justice Response.* Newbury Park, Calif.: Sage.

Cadsky, O., and M. Crawford
1988 Establishing batterer typologies in a clinical sample of men who

assault their female partners. *Canadian Journal of Community Health* 7:119-127.

Caesar, P.L., and L.K. Hamberger

1989 Introduction: Brief historical overview of interventions for wife abuse in the United States. In P.L. Caesar and L.K. Hamberger, eds., *Treating Men Who Batter: Theory, Practice, and Programs.* New York: Springer.

Calhoun, K.

1990 Lies, Sex, and Videotapes: Studies in Sexual Aggression. Presidential address, presented at the Southeastern Psychological Association, Atlanta, Georgia, March. Psychology Department, University of Georgia.

Campbell, J.C.

1992 Wife-battering: Cultural contexts versus Western social sciences. Pp. 229-249 in D.A. Counts, J.K. Brown, and J.C. Campbell, eds., *Sanctions and Sanctuary: Cultural Perspectives on the Beating of Wives.* Boulder, Colo.: Westview Press.

Cannon, J.B., and J.S. Sparks

1989 Shelters—an alternative to violence: A psychosocial case study. *Journal of Community Psychology* 17:203-213.

Cazenave, N.A., and M.A. Straus

1990 Race, class, network embeddedness, and family violence: A search for potent support systems. Pp. 321-329 in M.A. Straus and R.J. Gelles, eds., *Physical Violence in American Families: Risk Factors and Adaptations to Violence in 8,145 Families.* New Brunswick, N.J.: Transaction Publishers

Centers for Disease Control and Prevention

1995 Summary of CDC's Program to Prevent Violence Against Women. Paper presented to the National Research Council's Committee on the Assessment of Family Violence Interventions, February 27-29, Washington, D.C.

Chappell, D.

1984 The impact of rape legislation reform: Some comparative trends. *International Journal of Women's Studies* 7:70-80.

Chester, B., R.W. Robin, M.P. Koss, J. Lopez, and D. Goldman

1994 Grandmother dishonored: Violence against women by male partners in American Indian communities. *Violence and Victims* 9(3):249-258.

Chin, K.

1994 Out-of-town brides: International marriage and wife abuse among Chinese immigrants. *Journal of Comparative Family Studies* XXV(1):53-69.

Christiansen, K.O.

1977 A review of studies of criminality among twins. In S.A. Mednick and K.O. Christiansen, eds., *Biosocial Bases of Criminal Behavior.* New York: Gardner.

Christopherpoulos, C., A.D. Cohn, D.S. Shaw, S. Joyce, J. Sullivan-Hanson, S.P. Kraft, and R.E. Emery
  1987 Children of abused women: I. Adjustment at time of shelter residence. *Journal of Marriage and the Family* 49:611-619.
Clark, R.D.
  1990 The impact of AIDS on gender differences in willingness to engage in casual sex. *Journal of Applied Social Psychology* 20:771-782.
Clark, R.D., and E. Hatfield
  1989 Gender differences in receptivity to sexual offers. *Journal of Psychology and Human Sexuality* 2:39-55.
Claussen, A.I.E., and P.M. Crittenden
  1991 Physical and psychological maltreatment: Relations among types of maltreatment. *Child Abuse and Neglect* 15:5-18.
Cloninger, C.R., and I.I. Gottesman
  1987 Genetic and environmental factors in antisocial behavioral disorders. Pp. 92-109 in S.A. Mednick, T.E. Moffitt, and S.A. Stack, eds., *The Causes of Crime: New Biological Approaches*. New York: Cambridge University Press.
Cloninger, C.R., K.O. Christiansen, T. Reich, and I.I. Gottesman
  1978 Implications of sex differences in the prevalences of antisocial personality, alcoholism, and criminality for familial transmission. *Archives of General Psychiatry* 35:941-951.
Coccaro, E.F., L.J. Siever, H.M. Klar, and G. Maurer
  1989 Serotonergic studies in patients with affective and personality disorders. *Archives of General Psychiatry* 46:587-598.
Coleman, D.H., and M.A. Straus
  1983 Alcohol abuse and family violence. Pp. 104-124 in E. Gottheil, K.A. Druley, T.E. Skoloda, and H. M. Waxman, eds., *Alcohol, Drug Abuse, and Aggression*. Springfield, Ill.: Charles C Thomas.
Coleman, K.H.
  1980 Conjugal violence: What 33 men report. *Journal of Marital and Family Therapy* 6:207-213.
Collins, J.J.
  1986 The relationship of problem drinking to individual offending sequences. Pp. 89-120 in A. Blumstein, J. Cohen, J. Roth, and C. Visher, eds., *Criminal Careers and Career Criminals, Volume II*. Panel on Research on Criminal Careers, Committee on Research on Law Enforcement and the Administration of Justice, National Research Council. Washington, D.C.: National Academy Press.
Comstock, G., and H. Paik
  1990 The effects of television violence on aggressive behavior: A meta-analysis. Paper prepared for the National Research Council Panel on the Understanding and Control of Violent Behavior. S.I. Newhouse School of Public Communication, Syracuse University.
Conklin, J.E.
  1975 *The Impact of Crime*. New York: Macmillan.

Cook, P.J.
  1977   Punishment and crime: A critique of current findings concerning the preventive effects of punishment. *Law and Contemporary Problems* 41:164-204.

Cook, S.L.
  1995   Acceptance and expectation of sexual aggression in college students. *Psychology of Women Quarterly* 19:181-194.

Corcoran, K.J., and L.R. Thomas
  1991   The influence of observed alcohol consumption on perceptions of initiation of sexual activity in a college dating situation. *Journal of Applied Social Psychology* 21:500-507.

Council on Scientific Affairs, American Medical Association
  1992   Violence against women: Relevance for medical practitioners. *Journal of the American Medical Association.* 267(23):3184-3189.

Counts, D.A., J.K. Brown, and J.C. Campbell, eds.
  1992   *Sanctions and Sanctuary: Cultural Perspectives on the Beating of Wives.* Boulder, Colo.: Westview Press.

Cox, J.W., and C.D. Stoltenberg
  1991   Evaluation of treatment program for battered wives. *Journal of Family Violence* 6(4): 395-413.

Craig, M.E.
  1990   Coercive sexuality in dating relationships: A situational model. *Clinical Psychology Review* 10:395-423.

Crenshaw, K.
  1991   Mapping the margins: Intersectionality, identity politics, and violence against women of color. *Stanford Law Review* 43(6): 1241-1299.

Crowe, L.C., and W.H. George
  1989   Alcohol and human sexuality: Review and integration. *Psychological Bulletin* 105:374-386.

Daly, M., and M. Wilson
  1988   Evolutionary social psychology and family homicide. *Science* 242:519-524.

Darke, J.L.
  1990   Sexual aggression: Achieving power through humiliation. Pp. 55-72 in W.L. Marshall, D.R. Laws, and H.E. Barbaree, eds., *Handbook of Sexual Assault: Issues, Theories, and Treatment of the Offender.* New York: Plenum Press.

Davidson, J.R., and E.B. Foa
  1991   Diagnostic issues in posttraumatic stress disorder: Considerations for the *DSM-IV. Journal of Abnormal Psychology* 100:346-355.
  1993   *Posttraumatic Stress Disorder: DSM-IV and Beyond.* Washington, D.C.: American Psychiatric Press.

Davis, R., B. Taylor, and S. Bench
  1995   Impact of sexual and nonsexual assault on secondary victims. *Violence and Victims* 10(1):73-84.

Davis, R.C., and B.G. Taylor
  1995 Proactive Response to Family Violence: The Results of a Randomized Experiment. Unpublished manuscript. Victim Services, Research Division, New York City.
Davis, R.C., E. Brickman, and T. Baker
  1991 Supportive and unsupportive responses of others to rape victims: Effects on concurrent victim adjustment. *American Journal of Community Psychology* 19:443-451.
DeMaris, A., and J.K. Jackson
  1987 Batterers reports of recidivism after counseling. *Social Casework* 68(8):458-465.
D'Ercole, A., and E. Struening
  1990 Victimization among homeless women: Implications for service delivery. *Journal of Community Psychology* 18(2), 141-152.
Deschner, J.P., J.S. McNeil, and M.G. Moore
  1986 A treatment model for batterers. *Social Casework* 67:55-60.
Detre, T., D.J. Kupfer, and J.D. Taub
  1975 The nosology of violence. Pp. 294-316 in W.S. Fields and W.H. Sweet, eds., *Neural Bases of Violence and Aggression.* St. Louis: Green.
Dobash, R.E., and R. Dobash
  1979 *Violence Against Wives.* New York: Free Press.
  1992 *Women, Violence, and Social Change.* New York: Routledge.
Donnelly, D., and K. Cook
  1995 Racial Differences in Shelter Utilization in the Deep South. Paper persented at the 4th International Family Violence Research Conference, Durham, New Hampshire, July 21-24. Department of Sociology, Georgia State University.
Donnerstein, E., and D. Linz
  1994 Sexual violence in the mass media. Pp. 9-36 in M. Costanzo and S. Oskamp, eds., *Violence and the Law.* Newbury Park, Calif.: Sage.
Dryfoos, J.G.
  1991 *Adolescents at Risk.* New York: Oxford University Press.
Dunford, F.W., D. Huizinga, and D. Elliott
  1990 The role of arrest in domestic assault: The Omaha police experiment. *Criminology* 28(2):183-206.
Dunn, S.P., and V.J. Gilchrist
  1993 Sexual assault. *Primary Care* 20:3184-4169.
Dutton, D.G.
  1986 The outcome of court-mandated treatment for wife assault: A quasi-experimental evaluation. *Violence and Victims* 1:163-175.
  1988 *The Domestic Assault of Women: Psychological and Criminal Justice Perspectives.* Boston: Allyn and Bacon.
  1994 The origin and structure of the abusive personality. *Journal of Personality Disorders* 8(3):181-191.

1995   Trauma symptoms and PTSD-like profiles in perpetrators of intimate abuse. *Journal of Traumatic Stress* 8(2):299-316.

Dutton, D.G., and J.J. Browning
1988   Concern for power, fear of intimacy, and aversive stimuli for wife assault. Pp. 163-175 in G. Hotaling, D. Finkelhor, J.T. Kirkpatrick, and M.A. Straus, eds., *Family Abuse and Its Consequences: New Directions in Research.* Newbury Park, Calif.: Sage.

Dutton, D.G., and A.J. Starzomski
1993   Borderline personality in perpetrators of psychological and physical abuse. *Violence and Victims* 8(4):327-337.

Dutton, D.G., K. Saunders, A. Starzomski, and K. Bartholomew
1994   Intimacy-anger and insecure attachments as precursors of abuse in intimate relationships. *Journal of Applied Social Psychology* 24:1367-1386.

Dutton, M.A.
1992a *Empowering and Healing the Battered Woman: A Model for Assessment and Intervention.* New York: Springer.
1992b Assessment and treatment of PTSD among battered women. Pp. 69-98 in D. Foy, ed., *Treating PTSD: Cognitive and Behavioral Strategies.* New York: Guilford.
1993   Understanding women's responses to domestic violence: A redefinition of battered woman syndrome. *Hofstra Law Review* 21:1191-1242.

Dworkin, A.
1991   *Pornography: Men Possessing Women.* New York: NAL/Dutton.

Dye, E., and S. Roth
1990   Psychotherapists' knowledge about and attitudes toward sexual assault victim clients. *Psychology of Women Quarterly* 14:191-212.

Eaton, M.
1995   Lesbian Battering and Feminist Theories of Domestic Violence. Paper prepared for the Panel on Research on Violence Against Women. Columbia Law School, Columbia University.

Edleson, J.L., and M.P. Brygger
1986   Gender differences in reporting of battering incidents. *Family Relations* 35:377-382.

Edleson, J.L., and R.J. Grusznski
1989   Treating men who batter: Four years of outcome data from the Domestic Abuse Project. *Journal of Social Service Research* 12:3-22.

Edleson, J.L., and M. Syers
1990   The relative effectiveness of group treatments for men who batter. *Social Work Research and Abstracts* 26:10-17.

Edleson, J.L., and R.M. Tolman
1992   *Intervention for Men Who Batter: An Ecological Approach.* Newbury Park, Calif.: Sage.

Edleson, J.L., D.M. Miller, G.W. Stone, and D.G. Chapman
  1985 Group treatment for men who batter. *Social Work Research and Abstracts* 21:18-21.
Eisikovits, Z.C., and J.L. Edleson
  1989 Intervening with men who batter: A critical review of the literature. *Social Science Review* 63:384-414.
Elliott, C., L. Giddings, and A. Jacobson
  1985 Against no-drop policies. *NCADV Voice* (Summer).
Ellis, L.
  1989 *Theories of Rape: Inquiries into the Causes of Sexual Aggression.* New York: Hemisphere Publishing Co.
Epstein, J., and S. Langenbahn
  1994 The criminal justice and community response to rape. *Issues and Practices in Criminal Justice* May 1994. Washington, D.C.: National Institute of Justice, U.S. Department of Justice.
Eron, L.D.
  1982 Parent child interaction, television violence and aggression of children. *American Psychologist* 27:197-211.
Esbensen, F.A., and D. Huizinga
  1991 Juvenile victimization and delinquency. *Youth and Society* 23:202-227.
Essock-Vitale, S.M., and M.T. McGuire
  1985 Women's lives viewed from an evolutionary perspective. I. Sexual histories, reproductive success, and demographic characteristics of a random sample of American women. *Ethology and Sociobiology* 6:137-154.
Fagan, J.
  1996 The criminalization of domestic violence: Promises and limits. *NIJ Research Report* (January). Washington, D.C.: National Institute of Justice, U.S. Department of Justice.
Fagan, J., and A. Browne
  1994 Violence between spouses and intimates. Pp. 115-292 in A.J. Reiss, Jr., and J.A. Roth, eds., *Understanding and Preventing Violence: Vol. 3, Social Influences.* Panel on the Understanding and Control of Violent Behavior, Committee on Law and Justice, Naitonal Research Council. Washington, D.C.: National Academy Press.
Fagan, J., D.K. Stewart, and K.V. Hansen
  1983 Violent men or violent husbands? Background factors and situational correlates. Pp. 49-68 in D. Finkelhor, R.J. Gelles, G.T. Hotaling, and M.A. Straus, eds., *The Dark Side of Families: Current Family Violence Research.* Beverly Hills, Calif.: Sage.
Fagan, J., E. Friedman, S. Wexler, and V.L. Lewis
  1984 *National Family Violence Evaluation: Final Report. Volume 1: Executive Summary and Analytic Findings.* San Francisco: URSA Institute.
Fagot, B.I., R. Loeber, and J.B. Reid
  1988 Developmental determinants of male-to-female aggression. Pp.

91-105 in G.W. Russell, ed., *Violence in Intimate Relationships.* Costa Mesa, Calif.: PMA Publishng Corp.

Family Violence Prevention Fund
1995 Public concern about domestic violence is rising sharply, new poll finds, as more women say they have been abused. News release, August 16, San Francisco, Calif.

Farrington, D.P.
1991 Childhood aggression and adult violence: Early precursors and later-life outcomes. Pp. 5-29 in D.J. Pepler and K.H. Rubin, eds., *The Development and Treatment of Childhood Aggression.* Hillsdale, N.J.: Erlbaum.

Feazell, C.S., R.S. Mayers, and J. Deschner
1984 Services for men who batter: Implications for programs and policies. *Family Relations* 33:217-223.

Federal Bureau of Investigation
1991 *Uniform Crime Reports.* Washington, D.C.: U.S. Department of Justice.
1993 *Uniform Crime Reports.* Washington, D.C.: U.S. Department of Justice.

Ferraro, K.J.
1989 Policing woman battering. *Social Problems* 36:61-74.

Field, H.S.
1978 Attitudes toward rape: A comparative analysis of police, rapists, crisis counselors, and citizens. *Journal of Personality and Social Psychology* 36:156-179.

Figley, C.R., ed.
1985 *Trauma and Its Wake: The Study and Treatment of Posttraumatic Stress Disorder.* New York: Brunner/Mazel.

Fillmore, K.M.
1985 The social victims of drinking. *British Journal of Addiction* 80:307-314.

Fishbein, D.H.
1990 Biological perspectives in criminology. *Criminology* 28(1):27-72.

Fischer, K., and M. Rose
1995 When "enough is enough": Battered women's decision making around court orders of protection. *Crime & Delinquency* 41(4):414-429.

Fitzgerald, L.F.
1993 Sexual harassment: Violence against women in the workplace. *American Psychologist* 48:1070-1076.

Foa, E.B., G. Steketee, and B.O. Rothbaum
1989 Behavioral/cognitive conceptualizations of posttraumatic stress disorder. *Behavior Therapy* 20:155-176.

Foa, E.B., B.O. Rothbaum, D.S. Riggs, and T.B. Murdock
1991 Treatment of Posttraumatic Stress Disorder in rape victims: A comparison between cognitive-behavioral procedures and counseling. *Journal of Consulting and Clinical Psychology* 59:715-723.

Foa, E.B., B.O. Rothbaum, and G.S. Steketee
  1993 Treatment of rape victims. *Journal of Interpersonal Violence* 8(2):256-276.
Follingstad, D.R., L.L. Rutledge, B.J. Berg, E.S. Hause, and D.S. Polek
  1990 The role of emotional abuse in physically abusive relationships. *Journal of Family Violence* 5(2):107-120.
Follingstad, D.R., A.F. Brennan, E.S. Hause, D.S. Polek, and L.L. Rutledge
  1991 Factors moderating physical and psychological symptoms of battered women. *Journal of Family Violence* 6:81-95.
Ford, D.
  1983 Wife battery and criminal justice: A study of victim decision-making. *Family Relations* 32:463-475.
  1991 Prosecution as a victim power resource: A note on empowering women in violent conjugal relationships. *Law and Society Review* 25:313-334.
  1993 *The Indianapolis Domestic Violence Prosecution Experiment: Final Report.* Department of Sociology. Indianapolis, Ind.: Indiana University at Indianapolis.
Fortune, M.M.
  1983 *Sexual Violence: The Unmentionable Sin.* New York: Pilgrim Press.
Friedman, L.
  1995 Rethinking Social Services for Battered Women. Remarks presented at the Commonwealth Fund Symposium "Domestic Violence and Women's Health: Broadening the Conversation," New York, October. Victim Services, New York.
Friedman, L., and S. Couper
  1987 *The Cost of Domestic Violence: A Preliminary Investigation of the Financial Cost of Domestic Violence.* New York: Victim Services.
Friedrich, W.N., R.L. Beilke, and A.J. Urquiza
  1988 Behavior problems in young sexually abused boys: A comparison study. *Journal of Interpersonal Violence* 3:21-28.
Frieze, I.H., S. Hymer, and M.S. Greenberg
  1987 Describing the crime victim: Psychological reactions to victimization. *Professional Psychology* 18:299-315.
Frintner, M.P., and L. Rubinson
  1993 Acquaintance rape: The influence of alcohol, fraternity membership and sports team membership. *Journal of Sex Education and Therapy* 19:272-284.
Furby, L., M.R. Weinrott, and L. Blackshaw
  1989 Sex offender recidivism: A review. *Psychological Bulletin* 105:3-30.
Furby, L., B. Fischhoff, and M. Morgan
  1991 Rape prevention and self-defense: At what price? *Women's Studies International Forum* 14(1/2):49-62.

Gamache, D.J., J.L. Edleson, and M.D. Schock
1988 Coordinated police, judicial and social service response to woman battering: A multi-baseline evaluation across three communities. Pp. 193-209 in G.T. Hotaling, D. Finkelhor, J.T. Kirkpatrick, and M. Straus, eds., *Coping with Family Violence: Research and Policy Perspectives*. Newbury Park, Calif.: Sage.

Ganley, A.L., and L. Harris
1978 Domestic Violence: Issues in Designing and Implementing Programs for Male Batterers. Paper presented at the 86th Annual Convention of the American Psychological Association, Toronto, Ontario, Canada, August. Veterans Administration Hospital, Seattle, Wash.

Garner, J., J. Fagan, and C. Maxwell
1995 Published findings from the Spouse Abuse Replication Project: A critical review. *Journal of Quantitative Criminology* 11:3-28.

Garnets, L.D., and D.C. Kimmel, eds.
1993 *Psychological Perspectives on Lesbian and Gay Male Experiences*. New York: Columbia University Press.

Geerken, M.R., and W.R. Gove
1975 Deterrence: Some theoretical considerations. *Law and Society Review* 9:497-513.

Geffner, R., and A. Rosenbaum
1990 Characteristics and treatment of batterers. *Behavioral Sciences and the Law* 8:131-140.

Geller, J.A., and J. Walsh
1977- A treatment model for the abused spouse. *Victimology* 1:627-632.
1978

Gelles, R.J.
1988 Violence and pregnancy: Are pregant women at greater risk of abuse? *Journal of Marriage and the Family* 50:841-847.
1990 Methodological issues in the study of family violence. Pp. 17-28 in M.A. Straus and R.J. Gelles, eds., *Physical Violence in American Families: Risk Factors and Adaptations to Violence in 8,145 Families*. New Brunswick, N.J.: Transaction Publishers.

Gelles, R.J., and J.W. Harrop
1989 Violence, battering, and psychological distress among women. *Journal of Interpersonal Violence* 4:400-420.

Gelles, R.J., and M.A. Straus
1979 Determinants of violence in the family: Toward a theoretical integration. Pp. 549-581 in W.R. Burr, F.I. Nye, S.K. Steinmetz, and M. Wilkinson, eds., *Contemporary Theories About the Family*. New York: Free Press.

George, L.K., I. Winfield, and D.G. Blazer
1992 Sociocultural factors in sexual assault: Comparison of two representative samples of women. *Journal of Social Issues* 48:105-125.

George, W.H., K.H. Derman, G.L. Lehman, and A.M. Fors
1990 Alcohol Expectancy Set for Other and Perceived Sexual Disinhibi-

tion in a Live Analogue Interaction. Paper presented at the annual meeting of the Association for the Advancement of Behavior Therapy, San Francisco, California, November. W.H. George Department of Psychology, University of Washington.

George, W.H., K.L. Cue, P.A. Lopez, L.C. Crowe, and J. Norris
  1995 Self-reported alcohol expectancies and postdrinking sexual inferences about women. *Journal of Applied Social Psychology* 25:164-186.

Giacopassi, D.J., and R.T. Dull
  1986 Gender and racial differences in the acceptance of rape myths within a college population. *Sex Roles* 15:63-75.

Gibbs, J.P.
  1975 *Crime, Punishment, and Deterrence.* New York: Elsevier.

Gidycz, C.A., C.N. Coble, L. Latham, and M.J. Layman
  1993 Sexual assault experience in adulthood and prior victimization experiences: A prospective analysis. *Psychology of Women Quarterly* 17:151-168.

Gidycz, C.A., K. Hanson, and M.J. Layman
  1995 A prospective analysis of the relationships among sexual assault experiences. *Psychology of Women Quarterly* 19:5-19.

Gilbert, N.
  1995 Violence against women: Social research and sexual politics. Pp. 1-24 in Smith, M. D., D. J. Besharov, and K. N. Gardiner, eds., *Was It Rape! An Examination of Sexual Assault Statistics.* Meno Park, Calif.: The Henry J. Kaiser Family Foundation.

Giles-Sims, J.
  1983 *Wife Battering: A Systems Theory Approach.* New York: The Guilford Press.

Gilfus, M.E.
  1995 A Life-Span Perspective on Research on Violence Against Women. Paper prepared for the Panel on Research on Violence Against Women. Graduate School of Social Work, Simmons College.

Gilmartin-Zena, P.
  1987 Attitudes toward rape: Student characteristics as predictors. *Free Inquiry in Creative Sociology* 15:175-182.

Goldberg-Ambrose, C.
  1992 Unfinished business in rape law reform. *Journal of Social Issues* 48(1):173-185.

Golding, J.M.
  1994 Sexual assault history and physical health in randomly selected Los Angeles women. *Health Promotion* 13:130-138.

Golding, J.M., J.M. Siegel, S.B. Sorenson, M.A. Burnam, and J.A. Stein
  1989 Social support sources following sexual assault. *Journal of Community Psychology* 17:92-107.

Gomme, I.M.
  1986 Fear of crime among Canadians: A multivariate analysis. *Journal of Criminal Justice* 14:249-258.

Gondolf, E.W.

1985 Anger and oppression in men who batter: Empiricist and feminist perspectives and their implications for research. *Victimology* 10:311-324.

1987 Evaluating programs for men who batter: Problems and prospects. *Journal of Family Violence* 2(1):95-108.

1988 Who are those guys? Toward a behavioral typology of batterers. *Violence and Victims* 3:187-203.

1990 *Psychiatric Responses to Family Violence: Identifying and Confronting Neglected Danger.* Lexington, Mass.: Lexington Books.

1993 Treating the batterer. Pp. 105-118 in M. Hansen and M. Harway, eds., *Battering in Family Therapy.* Newbury Park, Calif.: Sage.

1995 Batterer Intervention: What We Know and Need to Know. Paper prepared for the Violence Against Women Strategic Planning Meeting, National Institute of Justice, Washington, D.C., March 31. Mid-Atlantic Addiction Training Institute, Indiana University of Pennsylvania.

Gondolf, E.W., and E.R. Fisher

1988 *Battered Women as Survivors: An Alternate to Treating Learned Helplessness.* Lexington, Mass.: Lexington Books.

Goodchilds, J., and G. Zellman

1984 Sexual signaling and sexual aggression in adolescent relationships. Pp. 233-243 in N. Malamuth and E. Donnerstein, eds., *Pornography and Sexual Aggression.* New York: Academic Press.

Goodchilds, J., G. Zellman, P.B. Johnson, and R. Giarrusso

1988 Adolescents and their perceptions of sexual interactions. Pp. 245-270 in A.W. Burgess, ed., *Rape and Sexual Assault.* New York: Garland.

Goolkasian, G.A.

1986 Confronting domestic violence: A guide for criminal justice agencies. *National Institute of Justice Issues and Practices.* May.

Gordon, M.T., and S. Riger

1989 *The Female Fear.* New York: The Free Press.

Gordon, R.

1983 An operational classification of disease prevention. *Public Health Reports* 98:107-109.

1987 An operational classification of disease prevention. Pp. 20-26 in J.A. Steinberg and M.M. Silverman, eds. *Preventing Mental Disorders.* Rockville, Md.: U.S. Department of Health and Human Services.

Gornick, J., M. Burt, and K. Pittman

1983 *Structure and Activities of Rape Crisis Centers in the Early 1980s.* Washington, D.C.: The Urban Institute

Grau, J., J. Fagan, and S. Wexler

1984 Restraining orders for battered women: Issues of access and efficacy. *Women and Politics* 4:13-28.

Greenblatt, C.S.
    1985 Don't hit your wife. . . unless: Preliminary findings on normative
          support for the use of physical force by husbands. *Victimology*
          10:221-241.
Greendlinger, V., and D. Byrne
    1987 Coercive sexual fantasies of college men as predictors of self-re-
          ported likelihood to rape and overt sexual aggression. *Journal of
          Sex Research* 23:1-11.
Griffin, S.
    1971 Rape: The all-American crime. *Ramparts* 10(September):26-36.
Grisso, J.A., A.R. Wishner, D.F. Schwarz, B.A. Weene, J.H. Holmes, and
R.L. Sutton
    1991 A population-based study of injuries in inner city women. *Ameri-
          can Journal of Epidemiology* 134(1):59-68.
Groth, A.N., and A.H. Birnbaum
    1979 *Men Who Rape: The Psychology of the Offender.* New York:
          Plenum.
Gwartney-Gibbs, P.A., J. Stockard, and S. Brohmer
    1983 Learning courtship violence: The influence of parents, peers, and
          personal experiences. *Family Relations* 36:276-282.
Hall, E.R., and P.J. Flannery
    1984 Prevalence and correlates of sexual assault experiences in adoles-
          cents. *Victimology* 9:398-406.
Hall, E.R., J.A. Howard, and S.L. Boezio
    1986 Tolerance of rape: A sexist or antisocial attitude. *Psychology of
          Women Quarterly* 10:101-118.
Hall, G.C.N.
    1990 Prediction of sexual aggression. *Clinical Psychology Review*
          10:229-245.
Hamberger, L.K., and J.E. Hastings
    1986 Personality correlates of men who abuse their partners: A cross-
          validational study. *Journal of Family Violence* 1:323-346.
    1989 Counseling male spouse abusers: Characteristics of treatment
          completers and dropouts. *Violence and Victims* 4:275-286.
    1991 Personality correlates of men who batter and non-violent men:
          Some continuities and discontinuities. *Journal of Family Vio-
          lence* 6:131-147.
    1993 Court-mandated treatment of men who assault their partner: Is-
          sues, controversies, and outcomes. Pp. 188-229 in N. Z. Hilton,
          ed., *Legal Responses to Wife Assault.* Newbury Park, Calif.: Sage
          Publications.
Hamberger, L.K., D.G. Saunders, and M. Hovey
    1992 The prevalence of domestic violence in community practice and
          rate of physician inquiry. *Family Medicine* 24:283-287.
Hampton, R.L., and R.J. Gelles
    1994 Violence toward black women in a nationally representative

sample of black families. *Journal of Comparative Family Studies* XXV(1):105-119.

Hanson, R.K.
1990 The psychological impact of sexual assault on women and children: A review. *Annals of Sex Research* 3:187-232.

Harrell, A.
1991 Evaluation of court-ordered treatment for domestic violence offenders. Washington, D.C.: The Urban Institute.

Harrell, A., B. Smith, and L. Newmark
1993 *Court Processing and the Effects of Restraining Orders for Domestic Violence Victims.* Washington, D.C.: The Urban Institute.

Harris, Louis and Associates
1993 *The Commonwealth Fund Survey of Women's Health.* New York: Commonwealth Fund.

Harris, R., S. Savage, T. Jones, and W. Brooke
1988 A comparison of treatments for abusive men and their partners within a family-service agency. *Canadian Journal of Community Mental Health* 7(2):147-155.

Hart, B.J.
1995 Coordinated Community Approaches to Domestic Violence. Paper presented at the Strategic Planning Workshop on Violence Against Women, National Institute of Justice, Washington, D.C., March 31. Battered Women's Justice Project, Pennsylvania Coalition Against Domestic Violence, Reading.

Hart, S.D., D.G. Dutton, and T. Newlove
1993 The prevalence of personality disorder among wife assaulters. *Journal of Personality Disorders* 7(4):328-340.

Hart, S.N., and M.R. Brassard
1991 Psychological maltreatment: Progress achieved. *Development and Psychopathology* 3:61-70.

Harvey, M.
1985 *Exemplary Rape Crisis Program: Cross-Site Analysis and Case Studies.* Washington, D.C.: National Center for the Prevention and Control of Rape. National Institute of Mental Health, National Institutes of Health, U.S. Department of Health and Human Services.

Hastings, J.E., and L.K. Hamberger
1988 Personality characteristics of spouse abusers: A controlled comparison. *Violence and Victims* 3(1):31-48.

Hazlewood, R.R., and A.W. Burgess, eds.
1995 *Practical Rape Investigation.* Boca Raton, Fla.: CRC Press.

Heise, L.L.
1993 Violence against women: The missing agenda. In M. Koblinsky, J. Timyan, and J. Gay, eds., *Women's Health: A Global Perspective.* Boulder, Colo.: Westview Press.

Heise, L.L., J. Pitanguy, and A. Germain
  1994 *Violence Against Women: The Hidden Health Burden.* World Bank Discussion Paper No. 255. Washington, D.C.: The World Bank.
Helton, A., J. McFarlane, and E. Anderson
  1987a Battered and pregnant: A prevalence study. *American Journal of Public Health* 77:1337-1339.
  1987b Prevention of battering during pregnancy: Focus on behavioral change. *Public Health Nursing* 4:166-174.
Hendricks-Mathews, M.K.
  1993 Survivors of abuse: Health care issues. *Primary Care* 20:391-406.
Herman, J.L.
  1986 Histories of violence in an outpatient population: An exploratory study. *American Journal of Orthopsychiatry* 56:137-141.
  1992 *Trauma and Recovery.* New York: Basic Books.
  1995 The Role of Psychological Abuse. Paper prepared for the NRC Workshop on Research on Violence Against Women, Washington, D.C., June 26-27. Department of Psychiatry, Harvard Medical School.
Herman, J.L., and Hirschman, L.
  1981 Families at risk for father-daughter incest. *American Journal of Psychiatry* 138:967-970.
Hilberman, E.
  1980 Overview: The "wife-beater's wife" reconsidered. *American Journal of Psychiatry* 137:1336-1347.
Hilberman, E., and K. Munson
  1978 Sixty battered women. *Victimology* 2:460-470.
Hindelang, M.J., M. Gottfredson, and J. Garofalo
  1978 *The Victims of Personal Crime .* Cambridge, Mass.: Ballinger.
Hindelang, M., T. Hirschi, and J.G. Weis
  1981 *Measuring Delinquency.* Beverly Hills, Calif.: Sage Publications.
Hirschel, J.D., I.W. Hutchison III, and C.W. Dean
  1992 The failure of arrest to deter spouse abuse. *Journal of Research in Crime and Delinquency* 29:7-33.
Ho, C.K.
  1990 An analysis of domestic violence in Asian American communities: A multicultural approach to counseling. *Women and Therapy* 9:129-150.
Holden, G.W., and K.L. Ritchie
  1991 Linking extreme marital discord, child rearing, and child behavior problems: Evidence from battered women. *Child Development* 62:311-327.
Holtzworth-Munroe, A.
  1992 Social skill deficits in maritally violent men: Interpreting the data using a social information processing model. *Clinical Psychology Review* 12:605-617.

Holtzworth-Munroe, A., and K. Anglin
  1991 The competency of responses given by maritally violent versus nonviolent men to problematic marital situations. *Violence and Victims* 6:257-269.
Holtzworth-Munroe, A., and G.L. Stuart
  1994 Typologies of male batterers: Three subtypes and the differences among them. *Psychological Bulletin* 116(3):476-497.
Horney, J., and C. Spohn
  1991 Rape law reform and instrumental change in six urban jurisdictions. *Law and Society Review* 25:117-153.
Hotaling, G.T., and D.B. Sugarman
  1986 An analysis of risk markers in husband to wife violence: The current state of knowledge. *Violence and Victims* 1:101-124.
Huston, A.C., E. Donnerstein, H. Fairchild, N.D. Feshbach, P.A. Katz, J.P. Murray, E.A. Rubinstein, B. Wilcox, and D. Zuckerman
  1992 Big world, small screen: The role of television in American society. Lincoln: University of Nebraska Press.
Institute of Medicine
  1994 *Reducing Risks of Mental Disorders: Frontiers for Preventive Intervention Research.* Washington, D.C.: National Academy Press.
Jaffe, P., S. Wilson, and D. Wolfe
  1986a Promoting changes in attitudes and understanding of conflict among child witnesses of family violence. *Canadian Journal of Behavioral Science* 18:356-380.
Jaffe, P., D. Wolfe, S. Wilson, and L. Zak
  1986b Similarities in behavior and social maladjustment among child victims and child witnesses to family violence. *American Journal of Orthopsychiatry* 56:142-146.
Jaffe, P., D. Wolfe., and S. Wilson
  1990 *Children of Battered Women.* Newbury Park, Calif.: Sage Press.
Jaffe, P.G., M. Sudermann, D. Reitzel, and S.M. Killip
  1992 An evaluation of a secondary school primary prevention program on violence in intimate relationships. *Violence and Victims* 7(2):129-146.
Jaffe, P.G., E. Hastings, D. Reitzel, and G.W. Austin
  1993 The impact of police laying charges. Pp. 62-95 in N.Z. Hilton, ed., *Legal Responses to Wife Assault.* Newbury Park, Calif.: Sage Publications.
Janoff-Bulman, R.
  1992 *Shattered Assumptions: Towards a New Psychology of Trauma.* New York: The Free Press.
Javorek, F.J.
  1979 When rape is not inevitable: Discriminating between completed and attempted rape cases for nonsleeping targets. *Research Bulletin* :75-82.

Jenny, C., T.M. Hooton, A. Bowers, M.K. Copass, J.N. Krieger, S.L. Hiller, N. Kiviat, and L. Corey
1990 Sexually transmitted diseases in victims of rape. *The New England Journal of Medicine* 322:713-716.

Johnson, J.D., and L.A. Jackson
1988 Assessing the effects of factors that might underlie the differential perception of acquaintance and stranger rape. *Sex Roles* 19:37-44.

Jones, L.E.
1991 The Minnesota School Curriculum Project: A statewide domestic violence prevention project in secondary schools. Pp. 258-266 in B. Levy, ed., *Dating Violence: Young Women in Danger*. Seattle, Wash.: Seal Press.

Joseph, J.
1995 Woman Battering: A Comparative Analysis of Black and White Women. Paper persented at the 4th International Family Violence Research Conference, Durham, New Hampshire, July 21-24. Criminal Justice Program, Stockton College of New Jersey.

Jouriles, E.N., and K.D. O'Leary
1985 Interspousal reliability of reports of marital violence. *Journal of Consulting and Clinical Psychology* 53:419-421.

Justice Research and Statistics Association
1996 *Report on State Domestic and Sexual Violence Data Collection*. Washington, D.C.: Justice Research and Statistics Association.

Kaftarian, S.J., and W.B. Hansen
1994 Improving methodologies for the evaluation of community-based substance-abuse prvention programs. CSAP Special Issue: Community Partnership Program. *Journal of Community Psychology* NSI:3-5.

Kagan, J.
1989 Temperamental contributions to social behavior. *American Psychologist* 44:668-674.

Kantor, G.K.
1993 Refining the brushstrokes in portraits on alcohol and wife assaults. Pp. 281-290 in *Alcohol and Interpersonal Violence: Fostering Multidisciplinary Perspectives*. NIAAA Monograph 24, NIH Publication No. 93-3496. Rockville, Md.: National Institute on Alcohol Abuse and Alcoholism, National Institutes of Health, U.S. Department of Health and Human Services.

Kantor, G.K., and J.L. Jasinski
1995 Prevention of Teen Dating Violence: Evaluation of a Multidimensional Model. Paper presented at the 4th International Family Violence Research Conference, Durham, New Hampshire, July 21-24. Family Research Laboratory, University of New Hampshire.

Kantor, G.K., and M.A. Straus
1987 The "drunken bum" theory of wife beating. *Social Problems* 34(3):213-230.

1990   The "drunken bum" theory of wife beating. Pp. 203-224 in M.A. Straus and R.J. Gelles, eds., *Physical Violence in American Families: Risk Factors and Adaptations to Violence in 8,145 Families.* New Brunswick, N.J.: Transaction Publishers.

Kantor, G.K., J.L. Jasinski, and E. Aldarondo
1994   Sociocultural status and incidence of marital violence in Hispanic families. *Violence and Victims* 9(3):207-222.

Katz, B.
1991   The psychological impact of stranger versus nonstranger rape on victims' recovery. Pp. 251-269 in A. Parrot and L. Bechhofer, eds., *Acquaintance Rape: The Hidden Crime.* New York: Wiley.

Kaufman, G.
1992   The mysterious disappearance of battered women in family therapists' offices: Male privilege colluding with male violence. *Journal of Marital and Family Therapy* 18:233-243.

Kellermann, A.L., and J.A. Mercy
1992   Men, women and murder: Gender-specific differences in rates of fatal violence and victimization. *Journal of Trauma* 33:1-5.

Kellermann, A.L., F.P. Rivara, N.B. Rushforth, J.G. Banton, D.T. Reay, J.T. Francisco, A.B. Locci, J. Prodzinski, B.B. Hackman, and G. Somes
1993   Gun ownership as a risk factor for homicide in the home. *New England Journal of Medicine* 329:1084-1091.

Kemp, A., E.I. Rawlings, and B.L. Green
1991   Posttraumatic stress disorder (PTSD) in battered women: A shelter example. *Journal of Traumatic Stress Studies* 4:137-148.

Kilpatrick, D.G., C.L. Best, L.J. Veronen, A.E. Amick, L.A. Villeponteaux, and G.A. Ruff
1985   Mental health correlates of criminal victimization: A random community sample. *Journal of Consulting and Clinical Psychology* 53:866-873.

Kilpatrick, D.G., B.E. Saunders, L.J. Veronen, C.L. Best, and J.M. Von
1987   Criminal victimization: Lifetime prevalence, reporting to police, and psychological impact. *Crime and Delinquency* 33:479-489.

Kilpatrick, D.G., C.N. Edmunds, and A.K. Seymour
1992   *Rape in America: A Report to the Nation.* Arlington, Va.: National Victim Center.

Kilpatrick, D.G., H.S. Resnick, B.E. Saunders, and C.L. Best
1994   Survey Research on Violence Against Women: Results from the National Women's Survey. Paper presented at the 46th annual meeting of the American Society of Criminology, November 11, Miami, Florida. National Crime Victims Research and Treatment Center, Medical University of South Carolina.

Kim, K., and Y. Cho
1992   Epidemiological survey of spousal abuse in Korea. In E. C. Viano, ed., *Intimate Violence: Interdisciplinary Perspectives.* Washington, D.C.: Hemisphere Publishing Corp.

Kimerling, R., and K.S. Calhoun
1994 Somatic symptoms, social support, and treatment seeking among sexual assault victims. *Journal of Consulting and Clinical Psychology* 62(2):333-340.

Kirchhoff, G., and C. Kirchhoff
1984 Victimological research in Germany—Victim surveys and research on sexual victimization. Pp. 57-64 in R. Block, ed., *Victimization and Fear of Crime: World Perspectives.* Washington, D.C.: U.S. Department of Justice, Bureau of Justice Statistics.

Klepper, S., and D. Nagin
1989 The criminal deterrence literature: Implications for research on taxpayer compliance. Pp. 126-155 in J.A. Roth and J.T. Scholz, eds., *Taxpayer Compliance. Volume 2: Social Science Perspectives.* Panel on Taxpayer Compliance Research, Committee on Research on Law Enforcement and the Administration of Justice, National Research Council. Philadephia: University of Pennsylvania Press.

Klodawsky, F., and C. Lundy
1994 Women's safety in the university environment. *Journal of Architectural and Planning Research* 11:2128-136.

Knickman, J.R., and B.C. Weitzman
1989 *A Study of Homeless Families in New York City: Risk Assessment Models and Strategies for Prevention. Final Report: Volume 1.* New York: Human Resources Administration, Health Research Program, New York University.

Knight, R.A., and R.A. Prentky
1990 Classifying sexual offenders. Pp. 23-52 in W.L. Marshall, D.R. Laws, and H.E. Barbaree, eds. *Handbook of Sexual Assault.* New York: Plenum.

Kochanek, K.D., and B.L. Hudson
1995 Advance report of final mortality statistics, 1992. *Monthly Vital Statistics Report* 43(6 Supplement, March 22):1-76.

Koretz, D.S.
1991 Prevention centered science in mental health. *American Journal of Community Psychology* 19(4):453-458.

Koss, M.P.
1985 The hidden rape victim: Personality, attitudinal, and situational characteristics. *Psychology of Women Quarterly* 9:193-212.
1988 Hidden rape: Sexual aggression and victimization in a national sample of students in higher education. Pp. 3-25 in A.W. Burgess, ed., *Rape and Sexual Assault, Vol. 2.* New York: Garland.
1990 The women's mental health research agenda: Violence against women. *American Psychologist* 45:374-380.
1992 The underdetection of rape: Methodological choices influence incidence estimates. *Journal of Social Issues* 48:61-76.
1993 Detecting the scope of rape: A review of prevalence research methods. *Journal of Interpersonal Violence* 8(2):198-222.

Koss, M.P., and T.E. Dinero
    1989 Discriminant analysis of risk factors for sexual victimization among a national sample of college women. *Journal of Consulting and Clinical Psychology* 57:242-250.
Koss, M.P., and J.A. Gaines
    1993 The prediction of sexual aggression by alcohol use, athletic participation, and fraternity affiliation. *Journal of Interpersonal Violence* 8:94-106.
Koss, M.P., and M.R. Harvey
    1991 *The Rape Victim: Clinical and Community Interventions.* Newbury Park, CA: Sage.
Koss, M.P., and L. Heslet
    1992 Somatic consequences of violence against women. *Archives of Family Medicine* 1:53-59.
Koss, M.P., and C. Oros
    1982 The sexual experiences survey: A research instrument investigating sexual aggression and victimization. *Journal of Consulting and Clinical Psychology* 50:455-457.
Koss, M.P., K.E. Leonard, D.A. Beezley, and C.J. Oros
    1985 Nonstranger sexual aggression: A discriminant analysis of the psychological characteristics of undetected offenders. *Sex Roles* 12:981-992.
Koss, M.P., C.A. Gidcyz, and N. Wisniewski
    1987 The scope of rape: Incidence and prevalence of sexual aggression and victimization in a national sample of higher education students. *Journal of Consulting and Clinical Psychology* 42:162-170.
Koss, M.P., T.E. Dinero, C.A. Seibel, and S.L. Cox
    1988 Stranger and acquaintance rape. *Psychology of Women Quarterly* 12:1-24.
Koss, M.P., P.G. Koss, and W. Woodruff
    1991 Deleterious effects of criminal victimization on women's health and medical utilization. *Archives of Internal Medicine* 151:342-357.
Koss, M.P., L. Goodman, A. Browne, L. Fitgerald, G.P. Keita, and N.F. Russon
    1994 *No Safe Haven.* Washington, D.C.: American Psychological Association.
Kowalski, R.M.
    1992 Nonverbal behaviors and perceptions of sexual intentions: Effects of sexual connotativeness, verbal response, and rape outcome. *Basic and Applied Social Psychology* 13:427-445.
    1993 Inferring sexual interest from behavioral cues: Effects of gender and sexually-relevant attitudes. *Sex Roles* 29:13-31.
Lacey, H.B.
    1990 Sexually transmitted diseases and rape: The experience of a sexual assault center. *International Journal of STD and AIDS* 1:405-409.

LaFree, G.
   1989 *Rape and Criminal Justice.* Belmont, Calif.: Wadsworth.
Lalumière, M.L., and V.L. Quinsey
   1994 The discriminability of rapists from non-sex offenders using
         phallometric measures: A meta-analysis. *Criminal Justice and
         Behavior* 21(1):150-175.
Landolt, M.A., M.L. Lalumière, and V.L. Quinsey
   1995 Sex differences and intra-sex variations in human mating tactics:
         An evolutionary approach. *Ethology and Sociobiology* 16:3-23.
Lang, A., D. Goeckner, V. Adesso, and G. Marlatt
   1975 Effects of alcohol on aggression in male social drinkers. *Journal of
         Abnormal Psychology* 84(5):508-518.
Langan, P.A., and C.A. Innes
   1986 *Preventing Domestic Violence Against Women.* Washington,
         D.C.: Bureau of Justice Statistics, U.S. Department of Justice.
Langevin, R.
   1983 *Sexual Strands: Understanding and Treating Sexual Anomalies
         in Men.* Hillsdale, N.J.: Erlbaum.
   1990 Sexual anomalies and the brain. Pp. 103-113 in W.L. Marshall,
         D.R. Laws, and H.E. Barbaree, eds., *Handbook of Sexual Assault:
         Issues, Theories, and Treatment of the Offender.* New York: Ple-
         num Press.
Langevin, R., J. Bain, M.H. Ben-Aron, R. Coulthard, D. Day, L. Handy, G.
Heasman, S.J. Hucker, J.E. Purins, V. Roper, A.E. Russon, C.D. Webster,
and G. Wortzman
   1985 Sexual aggression: Constructing a predictive equation. A con-
         trolled pilot study. Pp. 39-76 in R. Langevin, ed., *Erotic Prefer-
         ence, Gender Identity, and Aggression in Men: New Research
         Studies.* Hillsdale, N.J.: Lawrence Erlbaum.
Larrain, S.
   1993 *Estudio de Frecuencia de la Violencia Intrafamiliar y la Condición
         de la Mujer en Chile* (Study of the Frequency of Intrafamilial Vio-
         lence and the Condition of Women in Chile). Santiago, Chile:
         Pan-American Health Organization.
Lasley, J.R.
   1989 Drinking routines, lifestyles and predatory victimization: A causal
         analysis. *Justice Quarterly* 6:529-542.
Ledray, L.E., and S. Arndt
   1994 Examining the sexual assault victim: A new model for nursing
         care. *Journal of Psychosocial Nursing and Mental Health Ser-
         vices* 32(2):7-12.
Leonard, K.E.
   1993 Drinking patterns and intoxication in marital violence: Review,
         critique, and future directions for research. Pp. 253-280 in *Alco-
         hol and Interpersonal Violence.* Research Monograph-24, NIH
         Publication No. 93-3496. Rockville, Md.: National Institute on

Alcohol Abuse and Alcoholism, National Institutes of Health, U.S. Department of Health and Human Services.

Leonard, K.E., and H.T. Blane
1992 Alcohol and marital aggression in a national sample of young men. *Journal of Interpersonal Violence* 7(1):19-30.

Leonard, K.E., and T. Jacob
1988 Alcohol, alcoholism, and family violence. Pp. 383-406 in V.B. Van Hasselt, R.L. Morrison, A.S. Bellack, and M. Herson, eds., *Handbook of Family Violence*. New York: Plenum Press.

Lerman, L.G.
1981 Criminal prosecution of wife beaters. *Response to Violence in the Family* 4(3):1-19.
1986 Prosecution of wife beaters: Institutional obstacles and innovations. Pp. 250-295 in M. Lystad, ed., *Violence in the Home: Interdisciplinary Perspectives*. New York: Brunner/Mazel Publishers.

Levine-MacCombie, J., and M.P. Koss
1986 Acquaintance rape: Effective avoidance strategies. *Psychology of Women Quarterly* 10:311-320.

Levinson, D.
1989 *Family Violence in Cross-Cultural Perspective*. Newbury Park, Calif.: Sage.

Lewis, D.O., J.H. Pincus, M. Feldman, L. Jackson, and B. Bard
1986 Psychiatric, neurological, and psychoeducational characteristics of 15 death row inmates in the United States. *American Journal of Psychiatry* 143:838-845.

Lewis, D.O., J. Pincus, B. Bard, E. Richardson, L. Prichep, M. Feldman, and C. Yeager
1988 Neuropsychiatric, psychoeducational, and family characteristics of 14 juveniles condemned to death in the United States. *American Journal of Psychiatry* 145:584-589.

Lidberg, L., J.R. Tuck, M. Asberg, G.P. Scalia-Tomba, and L. Bertilsson
1985 Homicide, suicide and CSF 5-HIAA. *Acta Psychiatrica Scandinavica* 71:230-236.

Lieberman Research Inc.
1995 Domestic Violence Advertising Campaign Tracking Survey: Post-Wave 1—November 1994 to February 1995. Family Violence Prevention Fund, San Francisco, Calif.

Linnoila, M., J. DeJong, and M. Virkkunen
1989 Family history of alcoholism in violent offenders and impulsive fire setters. *Archives of General Psychiatry* 46:613-616.

Linnoila, M., M. Virkkunen, M. Scheinin, A. Nuutila, R. Rimon, and F.K. Goodwin
1983 Low cerebrospinal fluid 5-hydroxyindoleacetic acid concentration differentiates impulsive from nonimpulsive violent behavior. *Life Science* 33:2609-2614.

Linz, D., E. Donnerstein, and S. Penrod
    1988 The effects of long-term exposure to violent and sexually degrad-
          ing depictions of women. *Journal of Personality and Social Psy-
          chology* 55:758-768.
Linz, D., B.J. Wilson, and E. Donnerstein
    1992 Sexual violence in the mass media: Legal solutions, warnings,
          and mitigation through education. *Journal of Social Issues* 48:145-
          172.
Lisak, D.
    1994 Subjective assessment of relationships with parents by sexually
          aggressive and nonaggressive men. *Journal of Interpersonal Vio-
          lence* 9(3):399-411.
Lisak, D., and S. Roth
    1990 Motives and psychodynamics of self-reported, unincarcerated rap-
          ists. *American Journal of Orthopsychiatry* 60(2):268-280.
Loh, W.
    1980 The impact of common law and reform rape statutes on prosecu-
          tion: An empirical study. *Washington Law Review* 55:543-652.
Lonsway, K.A., and L.F. Fitzgerald
    1994 Rape myths: In review. *Psychology of Women Quarterly* 18:133-
          164.
Lore, R.K., and L.A. Schultz
    1993 Control of human aggression. *American Psychologist* 48:16-26.
Lurigio, A.J., and P.A. Resick
    1990 Healing the psychological wounds of criminal victimization: Pre-
          dicting postcrime distress and recovery. Pp. 51-67 in A.J. Lurigio,
          W.G. Skogan, and R.C. Davis, eds., *Victims of Crime: Problems,
          Policies, and Programs.* Newbury Park, Calif.: Sage.
Maguire, K., and A.L. Pastore, eds.
    1995 *Bureau of Justice Statistics Sourcebook of Criminal Justice Statis-
          tics-1994.* Report No. NCJ-154591. Washington, D.C.: U.S. Gov-
          ernment Printing Office.
Mahoney, E.R., M.D. Shively, and M. Traw
    1986 Sexual coercion and assault: Male socialization and female risk.
          Sexual Coercion and Assault 1:2-8.
Malamuth, N.M.
    1986 Predictors of naturalistic sexual aggression. *Journal of Personality
          and Social Psychology* 50(5):953-962.
Malamuth, N.M., and K. Dean
    1991 Attraction to sexual aggression. Pp. 229-248 in A. Parrot and L.
          Bechhofer, eds., *Acquaintance Rape: The Hidden Crime.* New
          York: Wiley.
Malamuth, N.M., R.J. Sockloskie, M.P. Koss, and J.S. Tanaka
    1991 Characteristics of aggressors against women: Testing a model us-
          ing a national sample of college students. *Journal of Consulting
          and Clinical Psychology* 59(5):670-681.

Malamuth, N. M., C.L. Heavey, and D. Linz
1993 Predicting men's antisocial behavior against women: The interaction model of sexual aggression. Pp. 63-97 in G.N. Hall, R. Hirschman, J. Graham, and M. Zaragoza, eds., *Sexual Aggression: Issues in Etiology, Assessment, and Treatment*. Washington, D.C.: Hemisphere.

Malamuth, N.M., D. Linz, C.L. Heavey, G. Barnes, and M. Acker
1995 Using the confluence model of sexual aggression to predict men's conflict with women: A ten-year follow-up study. *Journal of Personality and Social Psychology* 69(2):353-369.

Mann, J.D.
1987 Psychobiological predictors of suicide. *Journal of Clinical Psychiatry* 48:39-43.

March, J.S.
1990 The nosology of posttraumatic stress disorder. *Journal of Anxiety Disorders* 4:61-82.

Margolin, G., R.S. John, and L. Gleberman
1988 Affective responses to conflictual discussions in violent and nonviolent couples. *Journal of Consulting and Clinical Psychology* 56:24-33.

Margolin, L., M. Miller, and P.B. Moran
1989 When a kiss is not just a kiss: Relating violations of consent in kissing to rape myth acceptance. *Sex Roles* 20:231-242.

Marques, J.K., D.M. Day, C. Nelson, and M.A. West
1994 Effects of cognitive-behavioral treatment on sex offender recidivism: Preliminary results of a longitudinal study. *Criminal Justice and Behavior* 21(1):28-54.

Marshall, W.L.
1993 The treatment of sex offenders. *Journal of Interpersonal Violence* 8(4):524-530.

Marshall, W.L., and H.E. Barbaree
1990 An integrated theory of the etiology of sexual offending. Pp. 257-275 in W.L. Marshall, D.R. Laws, and H.E. Barbaree, eds., *Handbook of Sexual Assault: Issues, Theories, and Treatment of the Offender*. New York: Plenum Press.

Marshall, W.L., R. Jones, T. Ward, P. Johnston, and H.E. Barbaree
1991 Treatment outcome with sex offenders. *Clinical Psychology Review* 11:465-485.

Martin, D.
1976 *Battered Wives*. San Francisco: Glide.

McAfee, R.E.
1995 Physicians and domestic violence: Can we make a difference? *Journal of the American Medical Association* 273(22):1790-1791.

McCann, I.L., and L.A. Perlman
1990 *Psychological Trauma and the Adult Survivor: Theory, Therapy, and Transformation*. New York: Brunner/Mazel.

McCann, I.L., D.K. Sakheim, and D.J. Abrahamson
  1988 Trauma and victimization: A model of psychological adaptation.
        The Counseling Psychologist 6:531-594.
McFarlane, J., B. Parker, K. Soeken, and L. Bullock
  1992 Assessing abuse during pregnancy: Severity and frequency of inju-
        ries and associated entry into prenatal care. *Journal of the Ameri-
        can Medical Association* 267:3176-3178.
McGee, R.A., and D.A. Wolfe
  1991 Psychological maltreatment: Toward an operational definition.
        Development and Psychopathology 3:3-18.
McGrath, E., G.P. Keita, B.R. Strickland, and N.F. Russo, eds.
  1990 *Women and Depression: Risk Factors and Treatment Issues.*
        Washington, D.C.: American Psychological Association.
McKenry, P.C., T.W. Julian, and S.M. Gavazzi
  1995 Toward a biopsychosocial model of domestic violence. *Journal of
        Marriage and the Family* 57(May):307-320.
Mediascope
  1996 *National Television Violence Study: Executive Summary 1994-
        1995.* Studio City, Calif.: Mediascope, Inc.
Mednick, S.A., W.F. Gabrielli, and B. Hutchings
  1984 Genetic influences in criminal convictions: Evidence from an
        adoption cohort. *Science* 224:891-894.
Mercy, J.A., and L.E. Saltzman
  1989 Fatal violence among spouses in the United States, 1976-1985.
        American Journal of Public Health 79:595-599.
Meredith, W.H., D.A. Abbott, and S.L. Adams
  1986 Family violence: Its relation to marital and parental satisfaction
        and family strength. *Journal of Family Violence* 1:299-305.
Meyer, H.
  1992 The billion-dollar epidemic. *American Medical News*, January 6.
Miczek, K.A., A.F. Mirsky, G. Carey, J. DeBold, and A. Raine
  1994a An overview of biological influences on violent behavior. Pp. 1-20
        in A.J. Reiss, K.A. Miczek, and J.A. Roth, eds., *Understanding and
        Preventing Violence: Volume 2, Biobehavioral Influences.* Panel
        on the Understanding and Control of Violent Behavior, Commit-
        tee on Law and Justice, National Research Council. Washington,
        D.C.: National Academy Press.
Miczek, K.A., M. Haney, J. Tidey, J. Vivian, and E. Weerts
  1994b Neurochemistry and pharmacotherapeutic management of aggres-
        sion and violence. Pp. 245-514 in A.J. Reiss, K.A. Miczek, and J.A.
        Roth, eds., *Understanding and Preventing Violence: Volume 2,
        Biobehavioral Influences.* Panel on the Understanding and Con-
        trol of Violent Behavior, Committee on Law and Justice, National
        Research Council. Washington, D.C.: National Academy Press.
Miller, B.A.
  1992 Family Violence and Children: An Overview. Keynote address at
        the second annual Center for Education and Drug Abuse Research

Conference, Pittsburgh, Pennsylvania, February. Research Institute of Alcoholism, New York State Division of Alcoholism and Alcohol Abuse, Albany.

Miller, L.
1987 Neuropsychology of the aggressive psychopath: An integrative review. *Aggressive Behavior* 13:119-140.

Minnesota Higher Education Center Against Violence and Abuse
1995 *Responding to Violence and Abuse: Educating Minnesota Professionals for the Future.* Minneapolis: Minnesota Higher Education Center Against Violence and Abuse.

Minturn, L., M. Grosse, and S. Haider
1969 Cultural patterning of sexual beliefs and behavior. *Ethnology* 8:301-318.

Mirsky, A.F., and A. Siegel
1994 The neurobiology of violence and aggression. Pp. 59-172 in A.J. Reiss, K.A. Miczek, and J.A. Roth, eds., *Understanding and Preventing Violence: Volume 2, Biobehavioral Influences.* Panel on the Understanding and Control of Violent Behavior, Committee on Law and Justice, National Research Council. Washington, D.C.: National Academy Press.

Moore, K.A., C.W. Nord, and J.L. Peterson
1989 Nonvoluntary sexual activity among adolescents. *Family Planning Perspectives* 21:110-114.

Mosher, D.L., and R.D. Anderson
1986 Macho personality, sexual aggression, and reactions to guided imagery of realistic rape. *Journal of Research in Personality* 20:77-94.

Mrazek, P.J., and R.J. Haggerty, eds.
1994 *Reducing Risks for Mental Disorders: Frontiers for Preventive Intervention Research.* Committee on Prevention of Mental Disorders, Division on Biobehavioral Sciences and Mental Disorders, Institute of Medicine. Washington, D.C.: National Academy Press.

Muehlenhard, C.L., and M.A. Linton
1987 Date rape and sexual aggression in dating situations: Incidence and risk factors. *Journal of Counseling Psychology* 34:186-196.

Muehlenhard, C.L., D.E. Friedman, and C.M. Thomas
1985 Is date rape justifiable? The effects of dating activity, who initiated, who paid, and men's attitudes toward women. *Psychology of Women Quarterly* 9:297-310.

Muehlenhard, C.L., I.G. Powch, J.L. Phelps, and L.M. Guisti
1992 Definitions of rape: Scientific and political implications. *Journal of Social Issues* 48(1):23-44.

Mullen, P.E., S.E. Romans-Clarkson, V.A. Walton, and P.E. Herbison
1988 Impact of sexual and physical abuse on women's mental health. *Lancet* 1:841.

Mungas, D.
   1988 Psychometric correlates of episodic violent behavior: A multidi-
         mensional neuropsychological approach. *British Journal of Psy-
         chiatry* 152:180-187.
Muram, D., K. Miller, and A. Cutler
   1992 Sexual assault of the elderly victim. *Journal of Interpersonal Vio-
         lence* 7:70-77.
Murphy, C.M., and K.D. O'Leary
   1994 Research paradigms, values, and spouse abuse. *Journal of Inter-
         personal Violence* 9(2):207-223.
Murphy, S.M.
   1990 Rape, sexually transmitted diseases and human immunodeficiency
         virus infection. *International Journal of STD and AIDS* 1:79-82.
Murphy, W.D., E.M. Coleman, and M.R. Haynes
   1986 Factors related to coercive sexual behavior in a nonclinical sample
         of males. *Violence and Victims* 1:255-278.
Murray, J.P.
   1995 Children and television violence. *Kansas Journal of Law and Pub-
         lic Policy* 4(3):7-14.
Myers, M.P., D.L. Templar, and R. Brown
   1984 Coping ability of women who become rape victims. *Journal of
         Consulting and Clinical Psychology* 52:73-78.
National Institute of Mental Health
   1982 Television and Behavior: Ten Years of Scientific Progress and
         Implications for the Eighties (vol. 1), Summary Report. Rockville,
         Md.: National Institute of Mental Health, National Institutes of
         Health, U.S. Department of Health and Human Services.
   1992 Family Violence. National Workshop on Violence: Analyses and
         Recommendations. Report prepared by K.D. O'Leary and A.
         Browne. Rockville, Md.: Violence and Traumatic Stress Research
         Branch, National Institute of Mental Health, National Institutes
         of Health, U.S. Department of Health and Human Services.
National Institute of Justice
   1995 *Solicitation for Research and Evaluation on Violence Against
         Women.* Washington, D.C.: U.S. Department of Justice.
National Research Council
   1993 *Understanding Child Abuse and Neglect.* Panel on Research on
         Child Abuse and Neglect, Commission on Behavioral and Social
         Sciences and Education, National Research Council. Washington,
         D.C.: National Academy Press.
Neidig, P.H., D.H. Friedman, and B.S. Collins
   1985 Domestic conflict containment: A spouse abuse treatment pro-
         gram. *Social Casework* 66:195-204.
Nordby, V.
   1980 Reforming the rape laws: The Michigan experience. Pp. 3-34 in J.
         Scutt, ed., *Rape Law Reform.* Canberra: Australian Institute of
         Criminology.

Norris, F.H.
    1992 Epidemiology of trauma: Frequency and impact of different potentially traumatic events on different demographic groups. *Journal of Consulting and Clinical Psychology* 60:409-418.
Norris, F.H., and K. Kaniasty
    1991 The psychological experience of crime: A test of the mediating role of beliefs in explaining the distress of victims. *Journal of Social and Clinical Psychology* 10:239-261.
Norris, J., P.S. Nurius, and L.A. Dimeff
    1996 Through her eyes: Factors affecting women's perception of and resistance to acquaintance sexual aggression threat. *Psychology of Women Quarterly* 20(1):123-145.
Norton, I.M., and S.M. Manson
    1996 Research in American Indian and Alaska Native communities: Navigating the cultural universe of values and process. *Journal of Consulting and Clinical Psychology* 64(5).
    1997 Domestic violence intervention in an urban Indian health center. *Community Mental Health Journal* 33(4).
Nurius, P.S., and J. Norris
    1996 A cognitive ecological model of women's response to male sexual aggression in dating and courtship. *Journal of Psychology and Human Sexuality* 8(1/2).
Okun, L.
    1986 *Women Abuse: Facts Replacing Myths*. Albany: State University of New York Press.
O'Leary, K.D.
    1988 Physical aggression between spouses: A social learning theory perspective. Pp. 11-55 in V.B. Van Hasselt, R.L. Morrison, A.S. Bellack, and M. Hersen, eds., *Handbook of Family Violence*. New York: Plenum.
O'Leary, K.D., and I. Arias
    1988 Prevalence, correlates and development of spouse abuse. In R.D. Peters and R.J. McMahon, eds., *Social Learning and Systems Approaches to Marriage and the Family*. New York: Brunner/Mazel.
O'Leary, K.D., and A.D. Curley
    1986 Assertion and family violence: Correlates of spouse abuse. *Journal of Marital and Family Therapy* 12:281-289.
O'Leary, K.D., J. Malone, and A. Tyree
    1994 Physical aggression in early marriage: Pre-relationship and relationship effects. *Journal of Consulting and Clinical Psychology* 62:594-602.
O'Leary, K.D., R.E. Heyman, and P.H. Neidig
    1995 An Empirical Comparison of Physical Aggression Couples Treatment vs. Gender-Specific Treatment. Paper presented at the 4th International Family Violence Research Conference, Durham, New Hampshire, July 21-24. Department of Psychology, State University of New York at Stony Brook.

O'Sullivan, C., J. Wise, and V. Douglass
  1995 Domestic Violence Shelter Residents in New York City: Profile, Needs, and Alternatives to Shelter. Paper presented at the 4th International Family Violence Research Conference, Durham, New Hampshire, July 21-24. Victim Services, New York.

O'Sullivan, E.
  1976 What has happened to rape crisis centers? A look at their structures, members, and funding. *Victimology* 3(1-2):45-62.

Pagelow, M.D.
  1984 *Family Violence.* New York: Prager.
  1988 Marital rape. Pp. 207-232 in V.B. Van Hasselt, R.L. Morrison, A.S. Bellack, and M. Hersen, eds., *Handbook of Family Violence.* New York: Plenum Press.

Paik, H., and G. Comstock
  1994 The effects of television violence on antisocial behavior: A meta-analysis. *Communication Research* 21(4):516-546.

Palmer, S.E., R.A. Brown, and M.E. Barrera
  1992 Group treatment program for abusive husbands: Long term evaluation. *American Journal of Orthopsychiatry* 62(2):276-283.

Pan, H.S., P.H. Neidig, and K.D. O'Leary
  1994 Predicting mild and severe husband-to-wife physical aggression. *Journal of Consulting and Clinical Psychology* 62(5):975-981.

Paone, D., W. Chavkin, I. Willets, P. Friedman, and D. Des Jarlais
  1992 The impact of sexual abuse: Implications for drug treatment. *Journal of Women's Health* 1:149-153.

Pate, A.M., and E.E. Hamilton
  1992 Formal and informal deterrents to domestic violence: The Dade County spouse assault experiment. *American Sociological Review* 57:691-697.

Paternoster, R.
  1987 The deterrent effect of the perceived certainty and severity of punishment: A review of the evidence and issues. *Justice Quarterly* 4(2):101-146.

Paveza, G.
  1988 Risk factors in father-daughter child sexual abuse: A case-controlled study. *Journal of Interpersonal Violence* 3(3):290-306.

Pence, E., and M. Paymar
  1993 *Education Groups for Men Who Batter: The Duluth Model.* New York: Springer.

Pernanen, K.
  1976 Alcohol and crimes of violence. In B. Kissin and H. Begleiter, *The Biology of Alcoholism, Vol. 4.* New York: Plenum.

Pirog-Good, M., and J. Stets-Kealey
  1985 Male batterers and battering prevention programs: A national survey. *Response* 8:8-12.

Pittman, N.E., and R.G. Taylor
1992 MMPI profiles of partners of incestuous sexual offenders and part-
ners of alcoholics. *Family Dynamics of Addiction Quarterly* 2:52-
59.
Pleck, E.
1989 Criminal approaches to family violence, 1640-1980. Pp. 19-58 in
L. Ohlin and M. Tonry, eds., *Family Violence, Vol. 11: Crime and
Justice: An Annual Review of Research*. Chicago: University of
Chicago Press.
Plichta, S.B.
1995 Domestic Violence: Building Paths for Women to Travel to Free-
dom and Safety. Paper presented at the Symposium on Domestic
Violence and Women's Health: Broadening the Conversation, the
Commonwealth Fund, New York, September. College of Health
Sciences, Old Dominion University.
Plomin, R.
1989 Environment and genes. *American Psychologist* 44(2):105-111.
Prentky, R.A.
1990 Sexual Violence. Paper prepared for the National Research Coun-
cil Panel on the Understanding and Control of Violent Behavior.
J.J. Peters Institute, Philadelphia, Penn.
Prentky, R.A., and R.A. Knight
1991 Identifying critical dimensions for discriminating among rapists.
Journal of Consulting and Clinical Psychology 59(5):643-661.
PROFAMILIA
1990 *Encuestra de Prevalencia, Demografia y Salud* (Demographic and
Health Survey). Bogatá, Columbia: PROFAMILIA.
Ptacek, J.
1988 Why do men batter their wives? Pp. 133-157 in K. Yllö and M.
Bograd, eds., *Feminist Perspectives on Wife Abuse*. Beverly Hills,
Calif.: Sage.
Purdy, F., and N. Nickle
1981 Practice principles for working with groups of men who batter.
Social Work with Groups 4:111-122.
Quinsey, V.L.
1984 Sexual aggression: Studies of offenders against women. Pp. 84-
121 in D. Weistub, ed., *Law and Mental Health: International
Perspectives, Vol. 1*. New York: Pergamon.
Quinsey, V.L., and M.L. Lalumière
1995 Evolutionary perspectives on sexual offending. *Sexual Abuse*
7(4):301-315.
Quinsey, V.L., and D. Upfold
1985 Rape completion and victim injury as a function of female resistance strategy. *Canadian Journal of Behavioral Science* 17:40-50.
Quinsey, V.L., L.S. Arnold, and M.G. Pruesse
1980 MMPI profiles of men referred for pre-trial psychiatric assessment

as a function of offense type. *Journal of Clinical Psychology* 36:410-417.

Quinsey, V.L., G.T. Harris, M.E. Rice, and M.L. LaLumière
1993 Assessing treatment efficacy in outcome studies of sex offenders. *Journal of Interpersonal Violence* 8:512-523.

Quinsey, V.L., M.E. Rice, and G.T. Harris
1995 Actuarial prediction of sexual recidivism. *Journal of Interpersonal Violence* 10(1):85-105.

Radloff, L.S.
1977 The CES-D Scale: A self-report depression scale for research in the general population. *Applied Psychological Measurement* 1:385-401.

Raine, A., and P.H. Venables
1988 Skin conductance responsivity in psychopaths to orienting, defensive, and consonant-vowel stimuli. *Journal of Psychophysiology* 2:221-225.

Raine, A., P.H. Venables, and M. Williams
1990 Relationships between CNS and ANS measures of arousal at age 15 and criminality at age 24. *Archives of General Psychiatry* 47:1003-1007.

Randall, T.
1990 Domestic violence intervention calls for more than treating injuries. *Journal of the American Medical Association* 264:939-944.

Rapaport, K.R.., and B.R. Burkhart
1984 Personality and attitudinal characteristics of sexually coercive college males. *Journal of Abnormal Psychology* 93:216-221.

Rapaport, K.R., and D.D. Posey
1991 Sexually coercive college males. Pp. 217-228 in A. Parrot and L. Bechhofer, eds., *Acquaintance Rape: The Hidden Crime.* New York: Wiley.

Reilly, M.E., B. Lott, D. Caldwell, and L. DeLuca
1992 Tolerance for sexual harassment related to self-reported sexual victimization. *Gender and Society* 6:122-138.

Reiss, A.J., Jr., and J.A. Roth, eds.
1993 *Understanding and Preventing Violence.* Panel on the Understanding and Control of Violent Behavior, Committee on Law and Justice, National Research Council. Washington, D.C.: National Academy Press.

Resick, P.A.
1987 Psychological effects of victimization: Implications for the criminal justice system. *Crime and Delinquency* 33:468-478.
1990 Victims of sexual assault. Pp. 69-85 in A.J. Lurigio, W.G. Skogan, and R.C. Davis, eds., *Victims of Crime: Problems, Policies, and Programs.* Newbury Park, Calif.: Sage.

Resick, P.A., and M.K. Schnicke
1992 Cognitive processing therapy for sexual assault victims. *Journal of Consulting and Clinical Psychology* 60:748-756.

Resick, P.A., K.S. Calhoun, B.M. Atkeson, and E.M. Ellis
  1981 Social adjustment in victims of sexual assault. *Journal of Consulting and Clinical Psychology* 49:705-712.
Resick, P.A., C.G. Jordan, S.A. Girelli, C.K. Hutter, and S. Marhoefer-Dvorak
  1988 A comparative outcome study of behavioral group therapy for sexual assault victims. *Behavior Therapy* 19:385-401.
Richardson, D.R., and G.S. Hammock
  1991 Alcohol and acquaintance rape. Pp. 83-95 in A. Parrot and L. Bechhofer, eds., *Acquaintance Rape: The Hidden Crime.* New York: Wiley.
Riger, S., and M. Gordon
  1981 The fear of rape: A study of social control. *Journal of Social Issues* 37(4):71-92.
Riger, S., R.K. LeBailly, and M.T. Gordon
  1981 Community ties and urbanites fear of crime: An ecological investigation. *American Journal of Community Psychology* 9:653-665.
Riggs, D.S., and K.D. O'Leary
  1989 A theoretical model of courtship aggression. Pp. 53-71 in M. Pirog-Good and J.E. Stets, eds., *Violence in Dating Relationships.* New York: Praeger.
Rosenbaum, A.
  1986 Of men, macho, and marital violence. *Journal of Family Violence* 1(2):121-130.
  1988 Methodological issues in marital violence research. *Journal of Family Violence* 3:91-104.
Rosenbaum, A., and S.K. Hoge
  1989 Head injury and marital aggression. *American Journal of Psychiatry* 146:1048-1051.
Rosenbaum, A., S.K. Hoge, S. Adelman, W.J. Warnken, K. Fletcher, and R. Kane
  1996 Head injury in partner-abusive men. *Journal of Consulting and Clinical Psychology* (in press).
Rosenfeld, B.
  1992 Court-ordered treatment of spouse abuse. *Clinical Psychology Review* 12:205-226.
Ross, V.M.
  1977 Rape as a social problem: A byproduct of the feminist movement. *Social Problems* 25:75-89.
Roth, S., and L. Lebowitz
  1988 The experience of sexual trauma. *Journal of Traumatic Stress* 1:79-107.
Rothbaum, B.O., E.B. Foa, D.S. Riggs, T. Murdock, and W. Walsh
  1992 A prospective examination of posttraumatic stress disorder in rape victims. *Journal of Traumatic Stress* 5:455-475.

Rozee, P.D.
　1993　Forbidden or forgiven? Rape in cross-cultural perspective. *Psychology of Women Quarterly* 17:499-514.
Ruch, L.O., and S.M. Chandler
　1983　Sexual assault trauma during the acute phase: An exploratory model and multivariate analysis. *Journal of Health and Social Behavior* 24: 174-185.
Ruch, L.O., and J.J. Leon
　1983　Sexual assault trauma and trauma change. *Women and Health* 8:5-21.
Ruch, L.O., J.W. Gartrell, S. Armedeo, and B.J. Coyne
　1991　The sexual assault symptom scale: Measuring self-reported sexual assault trauma in the emergency room. *Psychological Assessment* 3:3-8.
Russell, D.E.H.
　1982　The prevalence and incidence of forcible rape of females. *Victimology* 7:81-93.
　1984　*Sexual Exploitation: Rape, Child Sexual Abuse, and Workplace Harassment.* Beverly Hills, Calif.: Sage.
　1989　Sexism, violence, and the nuclear mentality. Pp. 63-73 in *Exposing Nuclear Phallacies, 1st ed.* New York: Pergamon.
　1991　Wife rape. Pp. 129-139 in A. Parrot and L. Bechhofer, eds., *Acquaintance Rape: The Hidden Crime.* New York: John Wiley & Sons.
　1993　*Against Pornography: The Evidence of Harm.* Berkeley, Calif.: Russell Publications.
Sabourin, T.C., D.A. Infante, and J.E. Rudd
　1993　Verbal aggression in marriages: A comparison of violent, distressed but nonviolent, and nondistressed couples. *Human Communication Research* 20:245-267.
Sales, E., M. Baum, and B. Shore
　1984　Victim readjustment following assault. *Journal of Social Issues* 37:5-27.
Sanday, P.R.
　1981　The socio-cultural context of rape: A cross-cultural study. *Journal of Social Issues* 37(4):5-27.
Saunders, D.G.
　1992　A typology of men who batter. *American Journal of Orthopsychiatry* 62:264-275.
　1994　Cognitive-Behavioral and Process-Psychodynamic Treatments for Men Who Batter: Interactions Between Offenders' Traits and Treatments. Paper presented at the Association for the Advancement of Behavior Therapy, November. Department of Social Work, University of Michigan.
Saunders, D.G., and J.C. Parker
　1989　Legal sanctions and treatment follow-through among men who

batter: A multivariate analysis. *Social Work Research and Abstracts* (September):21-29.

Schechter, S.
1982 *Women and Male Violence*. Boston: South End Press.

Schei, B., and L.S. Bakketeig
1989 Gynecological impact of sexual and physical abuse by spouse: A study of a random sample of Norwegian women. *British Journal of Obstetrics and Gynecology* 96:1379-1383.

Schoop, R.F., B.J. Sturgis, and M. Sullivan
1994 Battered woman syndrome, expert testimony, and the distinction between justification and excuse. *University of Illinois Law Review* 1994(1):45-113.

Schriver, J.M.
1995 *Human Behavior and the Social Environment: Shifting Paradigms in Essential Knowledge for Social Work Practice.* Needham Heights, Mass.: Allyn and Bacon.

Schulman, M.
1979 *A Survey of Spousal Violence Against Women in Kentucky.* Washington, D.C.: Law Enforcement Assistance Administration, U.S. Department of Justice.

Selkin, J.
1978 Protecting personal space: Victim and resister reactions to assaultive rape. *Journal of Community Psychology* 6:263-268.

Shepard, M.F., and J.A. Campbell
1992 The Abusive Behavior Inventory: A measure of psychological and physical abuse. *Journal of Interpersonal Violence* 7(3):291-305.

Sherman, L.W.
1992 *Policing Domestic Violence: Experiments and Dilemmas.* New York: Free Press.

Sherman, L.W., and R.A. Berk
1984 The specific deterrent effects of arrest for domestic assault. *American Sociological Review* 49(2): 261-272.

Sherman, L.W., J.D. Schmidt, D.P. Rogan, D.A. Smith, P.R. Gartin, G.E. Cohn, D.J. Collins, and A.R. Bacich
1992 The variable effects of arrest on criminal careers: The Milwaukee Domestic Violence Experiment. *Journal of Criminal Law and Criminology* 83:137-169.

Shields, N.M., and C.R. Hanneke
1983 Battered wives' reactions to marital rape. Pp. 131-148 in D. Finkelhor, R.J. Gelles, G.T. Hotaling, and M.A. Straus, eds., *The Dark Side of Families: Current Family Violence Research.* Beverly Hills, Calif.: Sage.

Shields, N.M., G.J. McCall, and C.R. Hanneke
1988 Patterns of family and nonfamily violence: Violent husbands and violent men. *Violence and Victims* 3:83-97.

Shotland, R.L.
   1992 A theory of the causes of courtship rape: Part 2. *Journal of Social Issues* 48:127-145.
Siddle, D.A.T., A.R. Nicol, and R.H. Foggit
   1973 Habituation and over-extinction of the GSR component of the orienting response in anti-social adolescents. *British Journal of Social and Clinical Psychology*12:303-308.
Siegel, J.M., S.B. Sorenson, J.M. Golding, M.A. Burnam, and J.A. Stein
   1989 Resistance to sexual assault: Who resists and what happens? *American Journal of Public Health* 79:27-31.
Skogan, W.G., and M.G. Maxfield
   1981 *Coping with Crime: Victimization, Fear and Reactions to Crime in Three American Cities.* Beverly Hills, Calif.: Sage.
Smith, M.D.
   1994 Enhancing the quality of survey data on violence against women: A feminist approach. *Gender and Society* 8(1):109-127.
Smith, S.J.
   1989 Social relations, neighborhood structure, and the fear of crime in Britain. Pp. 1-23 in D. Evans and D.T. Herbert, eds., *The Geography of Crime.* London, England: Croom-Helm.
Softas-Nall, B., A. Bardos, and M. Fakinos
   1995 Fear of rape: Its perceived seriousness and likelihood among young Greek women. *Violence Against Women* 1(2):174-186.
Sohn, E.F.
   1994 Antistalking statutes: Do they actually protect victims? *Criminal Law Bulletin* 30(3):203-241.
Sorenson, S.B.
   1996 Violence against women: Examining ethnic differences and commonalities. *Evaluation Review* 20:123-145.
Sorenson, S.B., and J.M. Golding
   1990 Depressive sequelae of recent criminal victimization. *Journal of Traumatic Stress* 3:337-350.
Sorenson, S.B., and A.F. Saftlas
   1994 Violence and women's health: The role of epidemiology *Annals of Epidemiology* 4:140-145.
Sorenson, S.B., and C.A Telles
   1991 Self-reports of spousal violence in a Mexican American and a non-Hispanic white population. *Violence and Victims* 6:3-16.
Sorenson, S.B., J.A. Stein, J.M. Siegel, J.M. Golding, and M.A. Burnam
   1987 The prevalence of adult sexual assault: The Los Angeles Epidemiologic Catchment Area project. *American Journal of Epidemiology* 126:1154-1164.
Sorenson, S.B., D.M. Upchurch, and H. Shen
   1996 Violence and injury in marital arguments. *American Journal of Public Health* 86:35-40.
Stark, E., and A. Flitcraft
   1988 Violence among intimates: An epidemiological review. Pp. 293-

317 in V.B. Van Hasselt, R.L. Morrison, A.S. Bellack, and M. Hersen, eds., *Handbook of Family Violence.* New York: Plenum Press.

Stark, E., A. Flitcraft, and W. Frazier
1979 Medicine and patriarchal violence: The social construction of a 'private' event. *International Journal of Health Services* 9:461-493.

Stark, E., A. Flitcraft, D. Zuckerman, A. Grey, J. Robison, and W. Frazier
1981 *Wife Abuse in the Medical Setting: An Introduction for Health Personnel.* Domestic Violence Monograph Series, No. 7. Rockville, Md.: National Clearinghouse on Domestic Violence. (Available from National Clearinghouse on Child Abuse and Neglect, U.S. Department of Health and Human Services.)

Statistics Canada
1994 *Family Violence in Canada.* Product No. 89-5410-XPE. Ottawa Canada: Canadian Centre for Justice Statistics, Statistics Canada.
1993 The Violence Against Women Survey. *The Daily: Statistics Canada*, November 18.

Steinman, M.
1990 Lowering recidivism among men who batter women. *Journal of Police Science and Administration* 17:124-132.

Sternberg, K.J., M.E. Lamb, C. Greenbaum, D. Cicchetti, S. Dawud, R.M. Cortes, O. Krispin, and F. Lorey
1993 Effects of domestic violence on children's behavior problems and depression. *Developmental Psychology* 29(1):44-52.

Stets, J.E., and M.A. Straus
1990 Gender differences in reporting marital violence and its medical and psychological consequences. Pp. 151-165 in M.A. Straus and R.J. Gelles, eds., *Physical Violence in American Families: Risk Factors and Adaptations to Violence in 8,145 Families.* New Brunswick, N.J.: Transaction Publishers.

Stewart, B.D., C. Hughes, E. Frank, B. Anderson, K. Kendall, and D. West
1987 The aftermath of rape: Profiles of immediate and delayed treatment seekers. *Journal of Nervous and Mental Disease* 175:90-94.

Storaska, F.
1975 *How to Say No to a Rapist and Survive.* New York: Random House.

Straus, M.A.
1979 Measuring family conflict and violence. The Conflict Tactics Scale. *Journal of Marriage and the Family* 41:75-88.
1986 The cost of intrafamily assault and homicide to society. *Academic Medicine* 62:556-561.
1990a Injury and frequency of assault and the "representative sample fallacy" in measuring wife beating and child abuse. Pp. 75-91 in M.A. Straus and R.J. Gelles, eds., *Physical Violence in American Families: Risk Factors and Adaptations to Violence in 8,145 Families.* New Brunswick, N.J.: Transaction Publishers.

1990b Measuring intrafamily conflict and violence: The Conflict Tactics Scales. Pp. 29-47 in M.A. Straus and R.J. Gelles, eds., *Physical Violence in American Families: Risk Factors and Adaptations to Violence in 8,145 Families.* New Brunswick, N.J.: Transaction Publishers.

1990c The Conflict Tactics Scales and its critics: An evaluation and new data on validity and reliability. Pp. 49-73 in M.A. Straus and R.J. Gelles, eds., *Physical Violence in American Families: Risk Factors and Adaptations to Violence in 8,145 Families.* New Brunswick, N.J.: Transaction Publishers.

Straus, M.A., and R.J. Gelles
1986 Societal change in family violence from 1975 to 1985 as revealed in two national surveys. *Journal of Marriage and the Family* 48:465-479.

1990 How violent are American families? Estimates from the National Family Violence Resurvey and other studies. Pp. 95-112 in M.A. Straus and R.J. Gelles, eds., *Physical Violence in American Families: Risk Factors and Adaptations to Violence in 8,145 Families.* New Brunswick, N.J.: Transaction Publishers.

Straus, M.A., and C. Smith
1990 Violence in Hispanic families in the United States: Incidence rates and structural interpretations. Pp. 341-367 in M.A. Straus and R.J. Gelles, eds., *Physical Violence in American Families: Risk Factors and Adaptations to Violence in 8,145 Families.* New Brunswick, N.J.: Transaction Publishers.

Straus, M.A., R.J. Gelles, and S. Steinmetz
1980 *Behind Closed Doors: Violence in the American Family.* Garden City, N.Y.: Anchor Press.

Sue, D.W., and D. Sue
1990 *Counseling the Culturally Different: Theory and Practice.* New York: Wiley.

Sugarman, D.B., and G.T. Hotaling
1989 Dating violence: Prevalence, context, and risk markers. Pp. 2-31 in M.A. Pirog-Good, and J.E. Stets, eds., *Violence in Dating Relationships.* New York: Praeger.

Sullivan, C.M., and W.S. Davidson II
1991 The provision of advocacy services to women leaving abusive partners: An examination of short-term effects. *American Journal of Community Psychology* 19(6): 953-960.

Sullivan, C.M., J. Basta, C. Tan, and W.S. Davidson II
1992 After the crisis: A needs assessment of women leaving a domestic violence shelter. *Violence and Victims* 7(3):267-275.

Sullivan, C.M., R. Campbell, H. Angelique, K.K. Eby, and W.S. Davidson II
1994 An advocacy intervention program for women with abusive partners: Six-month follow-up. *American Journal of Community Psychology* 22(1):101-122.

Syers, M., and J.L. Edleson
1992 The combined effects of coordinated criminal justice intervention in woman abuse. *Journal of Interpersonal Violence* 7:490-502.

Symons, D., and B. Ellis
1989 Human male-female differences in sexual desire. Pp. 131-146 in A.E. Rasa, C. Vogel, and E. Voland, eds., *The Sociobiology of Sexual and Reproductive Strategies*. London: Chapman and Hall.

Szinovacz, M.E.
1983 Using couple data as a methodological tool: The case of marital violence. *Journal of Marriage and the Family* 45:633-644.

Taylor, B.G.
1995 An Evaluation of the Domestic Violence Prevention Project. Internal report. Research Division, Victim Services, New York.

Taylor, J.W.
1984 Structured conjoint therapy for spouse abuse cases. *Social Casework* 65:11-18.

Temkin, J.
1987 *Rape and the Legal Process*. London, England: Sweet and Maxwell.

Tittle, C.R.
1980 *Sanctions and Social Deviance: The Question of Deterrence*. New York: Praeger.

Tolman, R.M.
1988 The initial development of a measure of psychological maltreatment of women by their male partners. *Violence and Victims* 4:159-178.
1990 The Impact of Group Process on Outcome of Groups for Men Who Batter. Paper presented at the European Congress on the Advancement of Behavior Therapy, Paris, September. School of Social Work, University of Michigan.

Tolman, R.M., and L.W. Bennett
1990 A review of quantitative research on men who batter. *Journal of Interpersonal Violence* 5:87-118.

Tolman, R.M., and G. Bhosley
1989 A comparison of two types of pregroup preparation for men who batter. *Journal of Social Service Research* 13:33-44.

Tolman, R.M., and J.L. Edleson
1995 Intervention for men who batter: A research review. Pp. 163-173 in S.M. Stith and M.A. Straus, eds., *Understanding Partner Violence: Prevalence, Causes, Consequences, and Solutions*. Minneapolis, Minn.: National Council on Family Relations.

Torres, S.
1991 A comparison of wife abuse between two cultures: Perceptions, attitudes, nature, and extent. *Journal of Mental Health Nursing* 12:113-131.

Tutty, L.M.
1995 The Efficacy of Shelter Follow-Up Programs for Abused Women.

Paper presented at the 4th International Family Violence Research Conference, Durham, New Hampshire, June 21-24. Faculty of Social Work, University of Calgary.

U.S. Attorney General's Task Force on Family Violence
1984 *Final Report.* Washington, D.C.: U.S. Department of Justice.

Ullman, S.E., and R.A. Knight
1991 A multivariate model for predicting rape and physical injury outcomes during sexual assaults. *Journal of Consulting and Clinical Psychology* 59:724-731.
1992 Fighting back: Women's resistance to rape. *Journal of Interpersonal Violence* 7:31-43.

Urquiza, A., and B.L. Goodlin-Jones
1994 Child sexual abuse and adult revictimization with women of color. *Violence and Victims* 9(3):223-232.

van der Kolk, B.A.
1987 *Psychological Trauma.* Washington, D.C.: American Psychiatric Press.
1994 The body keeps score: Memory and the evolving psychobiology of posttraumatic stress. *Harvard Review of Psychiatry* 1(5):253-265.

Van Dijk, J.J.
1978 Public attitudes toward crime in the Netherlands. *Victimology* 3:265-273.

Veronen, L.J., and D.G. Kilpatrick
1982 Stress Inoculation Training for Victims of Rape: Efficacy and Differential Findings. Paper presented at the 16th Annual Convention of the Association for the Advancement of Behavior Therapy, Los Angeles, California. National Crime Victims Research and Treatment Center, University of South Carolina.

Virkkunen, M., J. De Jong, J. Barko, F.K. Goodwin, and M. Linnoila
1989a Relationship of psychobiological variables to recidivism in violent offenders and impulsive fire setters. *Archives of General Psychiatry* 46:600-603.

Virkkunen, M., J. De Jong, J. Barko, and M. Linnoila
1989b Psychobiological concomitants of history of suicide attempts among violent offenders and impulsive fire setters. *Archives of General Psychiatry* 46:604-606.

Wadsworth, M.E.J.
1976 Delinquency, pulse rate and early emotional deprivation. *British Journal of Criminology* 16:245-256.

Waigant, A., D.L. Wallace, L. Phelps, and D.A. Miller
1990 The impact of sexual assault on physical health status. *Journal of Traumatic Stress* 3:93-102.

Waldo, M.
1986 Group counseling for military personnel who battered their wives. *Journal for Specialists in Group Work* 11:132-138.

Walker, L.E.
1979 *The Battered Woman.* New York: Harper and Row.

1984 *The Battered Woman Syndrome.* New York: Springer.

1991 Posttraumatic stress disorder in women: Diagnosis and treatment of battered woman syndrome. *Psychotherapy* 28:21-29.

1992 Battered woman syndrome and self-defense. *Notre Dame Journal of Law, Ethics, and Public Policy* 6:321-334.

1994 *Abused Women and Survivor Therapy.* Washington, D.C.: American Psychological Association.

Warr, M.

1985 Fear of rape among urban women. *Social Problems* 32:239-250.

Webster, D.W.

1993 The unconvincing case for school-based conflict resolution programs for adolescents. *Health Affairs* 12(4):126-141.

Whipple, V.

1987 Counseling battered women from fundamentalist churches. *Journal of Marital and Family Therapy* 13:251-258.

White, J.W.

In   Male violence toward women: An integrated perspective. In R.
press G. Geen and E. Donnerstein, eds., *Human Aggression: Theories, Research, and Implications for Policy.* Orlando, Fla.: Academic Press.

White, J.W., and M.P. Koss

1993 Adolescent sexual aggression within heterosexual relationships: Prevalence, characteristics, and causes. Pp. 182-202 in H.E. Barbaree, W.L. Marshall, and D.R. Laws, eds., *The Juvenile Sex Offender.* New York: Guilford Press.

Widom, C.S.

1989 Does violence beget violence? A critical examination of the literature. *Psychological Bulletin* 106:3-28.

Williams, J.E., and K.A. Holmes

1981 *The Second Assault: Rape and Public Attitudes.* Westport, Conn.: Greenwood Press.

Williams, K.R., and R. Hawkins

1989 Controlling male aggression in intimate relationships. *Law and Society Review* 23:591-612.

Williams, L.M.

1994 Recall of childhood trauma: A prospective study of women's memories of child sexual abuse. *Journal of Consulting and Clinical Psychology* 62(6):1167-1176.

Williams, O.J.

1992 Ethnically sensitive practice to enhance treatment participation of African American men who batter. *Families in Society* (December 1992):588-595.

1994 Group work with African American men who batter: Toward more ethnically sensitive practice. *Journal of Comparative Family Studies* 25(1):91-103.

1995 Treatment for African American men who batter. *CURA Reporter* 25(3):6-10.

Williams, O.J., and R.L. Becker
  1994 Domestic partner abuse treatment programs and cultural compe-
       tence: The results of a national survey. *Violence and Victims*
       9:287-295.
Windle, M.
  1994 Substance use, risky behaviors, and victimization among a U.S.
       national adolescent sample. *Addiction* 89:175-182.
Winfield, I., L.K. George, M. Swartz, and D.G. Blazer
  1990 Sexual assault and psychiatric disorders among a community
       sample of women. *American Journal of Psychiatry* 147:335-341.
Wolfe, D.A., L. Zak, S. Wilson, and P. Jaffe
  1986 Child witnesses to violence between parents: Critical issues in
       behavioral and social adjustment. *Journal of Abnormal Child Psy-
       chology* 14:95-104.
Women's AID Organization
  1992 Draft report of the National Study on Domestic Violence.
       Women's AID Organizatoin, Kuala Lumpur, Malaysia.
Wyatt, G.E.
  1992 The sociocultural context of African American and white Ameri-
       can women's rape. *Journal of Social Issues* 48:77-91.
Wyatt, G.E., and S.D. Peters
  1986 Issues in the definition of child sexual abuse in prevalence re-
       search. *Child Abuse and Neglect* 10:231-240.
Wyatt, G.E., and M. Riederle
  1994 Sexual harassment and prior sexual trauma among African-Ameri-
       can and White American women. *Violence and Victims* 9(3):233-
       247.
Wyatt, G.E., D. Guthrie, and C.M. Notgrass
  1992 Differential effects of women's child sexual abuse and subsequent
       sexual revictimization. *Journal of Consulting and Clinical Psy-
       chology* 60:167-173.
Yoshihama, M., and S.B. Sorenson
  1994 Physical, sexual, and emotional abuse by male intimates: Experi-
       ences of women in Japan. *Violence and Victims* 9(1):63-77.
Zimring, F., and G. Hawkins
  1971 The legal threat as an instrument of social change. *Journal of
       Social Issues* 27:33.

Appendices

Biographical Sketches

ANN WOLBERT BURGESS (*chair*) is chair of the Division of Psychiatric Mental Health Nursing of the School of Nursing at the University of Pennsylvania. She previously served on the faculties of Boston University and Boston College and is a clinical specialist in psychiatric nursing in Pennsylvania and Massachusetts. Her areas of expertise include victimology, rape trauma, child pornography, sex crimes against children, and posttraumatic stress disorder. She has served on several state and national commissions, studies, and task forces that addressed issues of violence against women and children, including the Advisory Committee to the National Center on Rape Prevention and Control, of which she was chair, and the U.S. Attorney General's Task Force on Family Violence. Burgess is a member of the Institute of Medicine. She serves as a member of the editorial boards of several journals, including the *Journal of Interpersonal Violence*, and she is the coauthor of several books and many articles on rape and sexual assault, including *The Victim of Rape: Institutional Reactions*. Burgess holds degrees from Boston University (Ph.D., B.S.) and the University of Maryland (M.S.)

EZRA C. DAVIDSON (*vice chair*) is professor and chair of the Department of Obstetrics and Gynecology at Charles R. Drew University of Medicine and Science and vice chair and professor in the Department of Obstetrics and Gynecology at the Center for Health Sciences at the University of California, Los Angeles. He has served on numerous committees, advisory boards, and task forces, including the Task Force on Meeting the Needs of Young Children of the Carnegie Corporation of New York, and the Advisory Committee on Infant Mortality to the Secretary of Health and Human Services, which he chaired. Davidson served as president of the American College of Obstetricians and Gynecologists in 1990-1991. He was elected to membership in the Institute of Medicine (IOM) in 1991 and has served on several IOM study committees. Davidson served in the U.S. Air Force before completing his residency at Columbia University at Harlem Hospital in New York. He holds degrees from Morehouse College (B.S.) and Meharry Medical College (M.D.)

MARK I. APPELBAUM is a professor in the Department of Psychology and Human Development at Peabody College of Vanderbilt University and director of the Vanderbilt University Quantitative Systems Laboratory. His current research is focused on longitudinal designs and methodology in the study of human development, application of multivariate techniques to the analysis of behavioral data, and methodology for large-scale, multisite longitudinal studies. In conjunction with his research on applying statistical methods to behavioral science, Appelbaum designed two computer programs, The Statistician's Toolbox and The IFEEL Scoring Program. He has previously been a member of the faculty at the University of North Carolina at Chapel Hill and the University of Haifa in Israel, and he is the founding editor of the journal *Psychological Methods*. Appelbaum holds degrees in chemistry from the Carnegie Institute of Technology (B.S.) and in measurement psychology from the University of Illinois (Ph.D.).

LUCY BERLINER is the director of research of the Harborview Sexual Assault Center at the Harborview Medical Center and clinical associate professor of social work at the University of Washington in Seattle. Her work has focused on the symptoms and treatment of sexually abused children and the punishment of perpetrators of sexual abuse. Berliner has served on national and state advisory boards, including the National Advisory Board of the National Resource Center on Child Sexual Abuse, the National Advisory Board of the Association for the Treatment of Sexual Abusers, the Advisory Board of the American Professional Society on the Abuse of Children, and the Advisory Committee on Crime Victims' Compensation of Washington State's Department of Labor and Industries. She is the author of many articles on child sexual abuse and has served on the editorial boards of the *Journal of Interpersonal Violence, Violence Update,* the *International Journal of Child Abuse & Neglect,* and the *Journal of Child Sexual Abuse.* Berliner holds degrees from Earlham College (B.A.) and the University of Washington in Seattle (M.S.W.).

KIMBERLE WILLIAMS CRENSHAW is a professor of law at the University of California, Los Angeles, where she teaches criminal law, civil rights law, constitutional law, and race and gender law. In 1995-1996 she is a visiting professor at Columbia Law School. She previously served on the faculty of the University of California, Irvine. She has written a number of articles on race and gender. Prior to her faculty career, she served as law clerk to the Honorable Shirley S. Abrahamson of the Wisconsin Supreme Court. Crenshaw was assistant to the legal team who represented Anita Hill in Senate Judicial Committee hearings in 1991. Crenshaw holds degrees from Cornell University (B.A.), Harvard University (J.D.), and the University of Wisconsin (LL.M.).

NANCY A. CROWELL (*study director*) is a staff officer with the Commission on Behavioral and Social Sciences and Education in the National Research Council/National Academy of Sciences. She serves on the staff for the Committee on Assessment of Family Violence Interventions, has organized a number of workshops for the Board on Children, Youth, and Families, and previously staffed National Research Council studies on risk communication and policy implications of greenhouse warming. Trained as a pediatric audiologist, Crowell worked in a demonstration project for preschool hearing impaired children and their families at Ball State University. She also worked on several political campaigns and for a political polling and consulting firm prior to joining the National Research Council staff. She holds degrees from St. Lawrence University (B.S.) in mathematics and French and from Vanderbilt University (M.A.) in audiology.

JEFFREY L. EDLESON is a professor at the University of Minnesota School of Social Work. He has conducted intervention research at the Domestic Abuse Project (DAP) in Minneapolis for the past 12 years and is the DAP's Director of Evaluation and Research. His research interests include domestic violence, programs for batterers, and program evaluation. Edleson is currently organizing the Minnesota Higher Education Center Against Violence and Abuse, a center funded by the Minnesota Legislature and focused on the development of professional training in the area of violence and abuse. He has provided technical assistance to domestic violence programs across North America as well as in Israel, Singapore, India, and Romania. Edleson has coauthored numerous articles and books, including *Intervention for Men who Batter: An Ecological Approach*. Edleson is an associate editor of *Violence Against Women* and on the editorial boards of several journals. Edleson holds degrees from the University of California, Berkeley (A.B.) and the University of Wisconsin (M.S.W. and Ph.D.)

DAVID A. FORD is chair of the Department of Sociology at Indiana University-Purdue University at Indianapolis. His primary research interest is in criminal justice interventions for domestic violence. Ford also has been extensively involved in the legal aspects of domestic violence issues, directing a training project on family violence for law enforcement officers and organizing and chairing the Indianapolis Mayor's Commission on Family Violence. He is also a member of the Municipal Court Emergency Temporary Protective Order Implementation Group and of the Marion County Domestic Homicide Review Group. Ford has written a number of articles on criminal justice interventions for domestic violence. Ford holds degrees from Oberlin College (B.A.), the University of Hawaii (M.A.), and the University of Pittsburgh (Ph.D.).

LUCY N. FRIEDMAN is the executive and founding director of Victim Services, a New York City not-for-profit organization established to help victims recover from crime and to prevent violence. Prior to founding Victim Services in 1978, Friedman was associate director of the Vera Institute of Justice. As a longtime advocate for victim rights, Friedman has written on various aspects of crime, its impact on victims and their families, and its treatment in the criminal justice system. Friedman serves on the New York State Permanent Judicial Commission on Justice for Children and has served on the National Research Council's Panel on the Understanding and Control of Violent Behavior, the Advisory Council of the New York State Crime Victims Board, and the Advisory Council of the New York State Department of Social Services. Friedman is a recipient of the Osborne Medal, the President's Crime Victim Service Award, and the Marjery Fry Award for Outstanding Services in Victim/Witness Assistance. She holds degrees from Bryn Mawr College (B.A.) and in social psychology from Columbia University (Ph.D.).

RICHARD B. IGLEHART is deputy district attorney in Alameda County, California. Previously, he served as chief counsel to the California Assembly Committee on Public Safety and chief assistant attorney general in the California Attorney General's Office. He has also been a member of the faculty of the Hastings School of Law in San Francisco and presents yearly lectures on recent developments in criminal law for the Continuing Education of the Bar. Iglehart chaired the California Attorney General's Commission on the Enforcement of Child Abuse Laws and Committees on Sentencing Reform and on Statewide Training of the California District Attorneys Association. Iglehart holds degrees from the University of California, Berkeley (B.S.), and from the University of Santa Clara School of Law (J.D.).

MARY P. KOSS is a professor in the Department of Family and Community Medicine at the University of Arizona College of Medicine and a certified psychologist. She has also served on the faculties of Kent State University and St. Olaf College. Koss has been studying rape and sexual assault since the late 1970s, and has authored numerous publications on rape and sexual assault. She cochaired the American Psychological Association's Task Force on Violence Against Women, which produced the book *No Safe Haven: Male Violence Against Women at Home, at Work, and in the Community.* She is an associate editor of *Violence and Victims* and is a consulting editor on several journals, including the *Journal of Clinical and Consulting Psychology.* Koss also serves on the national faculty of Women's Veterans' Health Programs and is a consultant to The World Bank and the United Nations Population Council on rape internationally. Koss holds degrees from the University of Michigan, Ann Arbor (A.B.), and the University of Minnesota (Ph.D.).

ILENA M. NORTON is assistant professor in the Department of Psychiatry at the National Center for American Indian and Alaska Native Mental Health Research at the University of Colorado Health Sciences Center in Denver. She is a practicing psychiatrist at Denver General Hospital; formerly, she was the hospital's director of psychiatric emergency services. She has been a consultant to the domestic violence program of the Denver Indian and Family Health

Services and has directed the Asian Pacific Development Center in Denver. Norton's research interests include mental health research and domestic violence in American Indian and Alaska Native populations. She holds degrees from Stanford University (B.A.) and from the Yale School of Medicine (M.D.).

SUSAN B. SORENSON is an associate professor in residence at the Department of Community Health Sciences and director of the Violence Prevention Research Center at the University of California, Los Angeles, School of Public Health. For over a decade, Sorenson has taught a graduate-level course on family and sexual violence at UCLA. She is also a licensed clinical psychologist in private practice in California. Her research interests include domestic violence, sexual assault, child homicide, and violence prevention. Sorenson has coauthored a number of articles on physical and sexual assault. She serves on the Attorney General's Policy Council on Violence Prevention for the California Department of Justice and on the editorial boards of the *Journal of Traumatic Stress*, the *Journal of Child Sexual Abuse*, and the *Journal of Consulting and Clinical Psychology*. Sorenson holds degrees from Iowa State University (B.S.), the Illinois Institute of Technology (M.S.) and the University of Cincinnati (Ph.D.).

SARA TORRES is an associate professor and chair of the Department of Community Nursing, College of Nursing and Health Professions, University of North Carolina at Charlotte. She previously served on the faculties of Florida Atlantic University and the University of South Florida. Her clinical experience includes serving as program director of adult and adolescent care at Charter Lane Hospital and as director of Mental Health Clinic and Day Treatment Center at Pilgrim State Psychiatric Center. Torres has done specialized research on domestic violence in the Hispanic community and has written and spoken extensively on the subject. Active on a national, state, and community level, she is a member of the Nursing Network on Violence Against Women, the Family Violence Prevention Fund's Advisory Committee, the Food and Drug Administration's Psychopharmacologic Drug Advisory Committee, the Center for Disease Control Advisory Committee for Injury Prevention and Control, the North Carolina Coalition Against Domestic Violence, and the Battered Women's Shelter Advisory Committee in Mecklenburg County, among many others. She has won numerous awards for her efforts with the Hispanic community, including the U.S. Surgeon General's Exemplary Service Award in 1993. Torres is a Lieutenant Commander in the U.S. Navy Reserves and the current president of the National Association of Hispanic Nurses. She holds degrees from the State University of New York at Stony Brook (B.S.), Adelphi University (M.S.), and the University of Texas (Ph.D.).

ELIZABETH M. WATSON is chief of police in Austin, Texas. Previously, she was with the Houston Police Department, beginning as a detective of homicide, burglary, and theft and ending as chief of police. Watson is a member of the Police Executive Research Forum and has served on the board of directors of the International Association of Chiefs of Police. She is on the editorial board of the *American Journal of Police*. Watson holds a degree from Texas Technological University (B.A.).

LINDA M. WILLIAMS is research associate professor at the University of New Hampshire Family Research Laboratory. Previously, she served on the faculties of Bermuda College in Devonshire, Bermuda, the University of Maryland, and Temple University. She has also been research director at the Joseph J. Peters Institute and research associate at the American Foundation Institute of Corrections. Her primary research interests include characteristics of families at risk for sexual abuse of children, memory for childhood trauma, child fatalities, and outcome studies of adults abused as children. Williams is coauthor of numerous articles and several books, including *Nursery Crimes: Sexual Abuse in Day Care* and *The Aftermath of Rape.* Williams is president of the American Professional Society on the Abuse of Children. She holds degrees from Beaver College (B.A.) and the University of Pennsylvania (M.A., Ph.D.).

Workshop Topics and Speakers

WORKSHOP ON VIOLENCE AGAINST WOMEN:
RESEARCH, PRACTICE, AND POLICY

National Research Council
Foundry Building
Washington, D.C.
June 26-27, 1995

MEASURING VIOLENCE AGAINST WOMEN:
EPIDEMIOLOGY AND DATA COLLECTION

Moderator:	Lucy Berliner, Harborview Sexual Assault Center
Speaker:	Dean Kilpatrick, Director, Crime Victims Research and Treatment Center, Medical University of South Carolina
Discussants:	Ronet Bachman, Bureau of Justice Statistics
	Linda Saltzman, Behavioral Scientist, National Centers for Disease Control and Prevention
	Susan Sorenson, School of Public Health, UCLA

THE ROLE OF PSYCHOLOGICAL ABUSE

Moderator:	Lucy Friedman, Victim Services
Speaker:	Judith Herman, Department of Psychiatry, Harvard University

Discussants: K. Daniel O'Leary, Distinguished Professor,
Department of Psychology, University of Stony
Brook
Carole Warshaw, Director of Behavioral Science,
Cook County Hospital
James Wright, Critical Incident Response Group,
FBI Academy

SEXUAL OFFENDERS AND BATTERERS

Moderator: Jeffrey Edleson, University of Minnesota
Speakers: Donald Dutton, University of British Columbia
Howard Barbaree, Clarke Institute of Psychiatry
Discussants: Neil M. Malamuth, University of California at Los
Angeles
Amy Holtzworth-Monroe, Indiana University
Oliver Williams, University of Minnesota

CULTURALLY SENSITIVE RESEARCH AND PRACTICE

Moderator: Kimberle Crenshaw, UCLA School of Law
Speaker: Lettie Lockhart, University of Georgia
Discussant: Robert Hampton, University of Maryland
Ilena Norton, University of Colorado Health
Sciences Center

COMMUNITY-BASED SERVICES

Moderator: David Ford, Indiana University-Purdue University
at Indianapolis
Speaker: Ellen Fisher, Texas Council on Family Violence
Discussants: Barbara Hart, Pennsylvania Coalition Against
Domestic Violence
Evelyn Tomaszewski, Victims Asistance Network,
Northern Virginia

LIFESPAN PERSPECTIVES ON
VIOLENCE AGAINST WOMEN

Moderator: Linda Williams, Family Research Laboratory,
University of New Hampshire
Speakers: Ann Burgess, School of Nursing, University of
Pennsylvania
Richard Gelles, Director, Family Violence
Research Program, University of Rhode Island
Patricia Resick, University of Missouri at St. Louis

RESEARCH, PRACTICE, AND POLICY

Moderator:	Mark Appelbaum, Vanderbilt University
Speaker:	John Briere, University of Southern California Medical School
Discussants:	Richard Gelles, Director, Family Violence Research Program, University of Rhode Island
	Anne Menard, Director, National Resource Center on Domestic Violence
	Ted Miller, National Public Services Research Institute

Index